This Cheese Journal Belongs To:

_____

Dedication

This book is dedicated to all the amazing Cheese Lovers (Turophiles) in the world.

You are my inspiration in producing books and I'm excited to be able to help in the planning of all parts of your cheese making or eating hobby!

How to Use this Extensive Cheese Journal:

The purpose of this ultimate cheese planner is to keep all your various cheese making and eating information, all cheesy thoughts organized in one easy to find spot.

Here are some simple guidelines to follow so you can make the most of using this book:

1. 1. The first cheese section is to write the "Name of Cheese and which Factory bought at" of your cheese sessions to keep track of each one tested.

2. Most ideas are inspired by something we have seen. Use the "Flavors" section to write down and actually check mark which one you like, add it in so you can track which cheese you liked only to be reminded later.

3. The "Rind" section is for you to detail out any outer shell of the cheese you need to remember or ones that you didn't really care for..... Don't worry, there will be more space for you to go in-depth of the type of Rind you liked as well.

4. Some ideas require giving them a 1-5 stars to sort them out, the "Rating Star" section is great for that. Just easily make a check mark or two.

5. The "Texture Meter" section is so you can visually track your preferences and be inspired to finish that particular cheese!

6. And finally the "Milk" section is for you to make a check mark which milk used you prefer and progressing towards your goals of eating lots of different types of cheeses....

Have fun!

NAME OF CHEESE _____

FACTORY _____

RIND
- [ ] BLOOMY
- [ ] WASHED
- [ ] NATURAL
- [ ] DRY
  - [ ] WHITE
  - [ ] SALTY
  - [ ] THICK
  - [ ] SOFT
  - [ ] HARD
  - [ ] FUZZY
  - [ ] GRITTY

ORIGIN _____

DATE _____

PRICE _____

FLAVORS
- [ ] SALTY
- [ ] SWEET
- [ ] CRYSTALLINE
- [ ] CRUMBLY
- [ ] SHARP/TANGY
- [ ] MILKY/LACTIC
- [ ] LEMON
- [ ] BUTTERY/CREAMY
- [ ] GRASSY
- [ ] ROBUST
- [ ] HERBAL
- [ ] SKINKY
- [ ] CARAMEL
- [ ] MOLDY/BLUE
- [ ] NUTTY
- [ ] EARTHY

MILK
- [ ] COW
- [ ] SHEEP
- [ ] GOAT
- [ ] RAW
- [ ] OTHER: _____
  _____
  _____

TEXTURE METER
- RUNNY
- SOFT
- SEMI-SOFT
- SEMI-FIRM
- FIRM
- HARD

NOTES
_____
_____
_____
_____
_____

RATING
☆ ☆ ☆ ☆ ☆

NAME OF CHEESE _____

FACTORY _____

RIND
- [ ] BLOOMY
- [ ] WASHED
- [ ] NATURAL
- [ ] DRY
  - [ ] WHITE
  - [ ] SALTY
  - [ ] THICK
  - [ ] SOFT
  - [ ] HARD
  - [ ] FUZZY
  - [ ] GRITTY

ORIGIN _____

DATE _____

PRICE _____

FLAVORS
- [ ] SALTY
- [ ] SWEET
- [ ] CRYSTALLINE
- [ ] CRUMBLY
- [ ] SHARP/TANGY
- [ ] MILKY/LACTIC
- [ ] LEMON
- [ ] BUTTERY/CREAMY
- [ ] GRASSY
- [ ] ROBUST
- [ ] HERBAL
- [ ] SKINKY
- [ ] CARAMEL
- [ ] MOLDY/BLUE
- [ ] NUTTY
- [ ] EARTHY

MILK
- [ ] COW
- [ ] SHEEP
- [ ] GOAT
- [ ] RAW
- [ ] OTHER: _____

TEXTURE METER
- RUNNY
- SOFT
- SEMI-SOFT
- SEMI-FIRM
- FIRM
- HARD

NOTES
_____
_____
_____
_____
_____
_____

RATING ☆☆☆☆☆

NAME OF CHEESE _____

FACTORY _____

RIND
- [ ] BLOOMY
- [ ] WASHED
- [ ] NATURAL
- [ ] DRY
  - [ ] WHITE
  - [ ] SALTY
  - [ ] THICK
  - [ ] SOFT
  - [ ] HARD
  - [ ] FUZZY
  - [ ] GRITTY

ORIGIN _____

DATE _____

PRICE _____

FLAVORS
- [ ] SALTY
- [ ] GRASSY
- [ ] SWEET
- [ ] ROBUST
- [ ] CRYSTALLINE
- [ ] HERBAL
- [ ] CRUMBLY
- [ ] SKINKY
- [ ] SHARP/TANGY
- [ ] CARAMEL
- [ ] MILKY/LACTIC
- [ ] MOLDY/BLUE
- [ ] LEMON
- [ ] NUTTY
- [ ] BUTTERY/CREAMY
- [ ] EARTHY

MILK
- [ ] COW
- [ ] SHEEP
- [ ] GOAT
- [ ] RAW
- [ ] OTHER: _____
  _____
  _____

TEXTURE METER
- RUNNY
- SOFT
- SEMI-SOFT
- SEMI-FIRM
- FIRM
- HARD

NOTES
_____
_____
_____
_____
_____

RATING ☆☆☆☆☆

NAME OF CHEESE _____

FACTORY _____

RIND
- ☐ BLOOMY ☐ WASHED ☐ NATURAL ☐ DRY
  - ☐ WHITE   ☐ SALTY   ☐ THICK
  - ☐ SOFT   ☐ HARD
  - ☐ FUZZY   ☐ GRITTY

ORIGIN _____

DATE _____

PRICE _____

FLAVORS
- ☐ SALTY
- ☐ SWEET
- ☐ CRYSTALLINE
- ☐ CRUMBLY
- ☐ SHARP/TANGY
- ☐ MILKY/LACTIC
- ☐ LEMON
- ☐ BUTTERY/CREAMY
- ☐ GRASSY
- ☐ ROBUST
- ☐ HERBAL
- ☐ SKINKY
- ☐ CARAMEL
- ☐ MOLDY/BLUE
- ☐ NUTTY
- ☐ EARTHY

MILK
- ☐ COW
- ☐ SHEEP
- ☐ GOAT
- ☐ RAW
- ☐ OTHER: _____
  _____
  _____

TEXTURE METER
- RUNNY
- SOFT
- SEMI-SOFT
- SEMI-FIRM
- FIRM
- HARD

NOTES
_____
_____
_____
_____
_____

RATING ☆☆☆☆☆

NAME OF CHEESE _____

FACTORY _____

RIND
- ☐ BLOOMY ☐ WASHED ☐ NATURAL ☐ DRY
  - ☐ WHITE ☐ SALTY ☐ THICK
  - ☐ SOFT   ☐ HARD
  - ☐ FUZZY   ☐ GRITTY

ORIGIN _____

DATE _____

PRICE _____

FLAVORS
- ☐ SALTY
- ☐ SWEET
- ☐ CRYSTALLINE
- ☐ CRUMBLY
- ☐ SHARP/TANGY
- ☐ MILKY/LACTIC
- ☐ LEMON
- ☐ BUTTERY/CREAMY
- ☐ GRASSY
- ☐ ROBUST
- ☐ HERBAL
- ☐ SKINKY
- ☐ CARAMEL
- ☐ MOLDY/BLUE
- ☐ NUTTY
- ☐ EARTHY

MILK
- ☐ COW
- ☐ SHEEP
- ☐ GOAT
- ☐ RAW
- ☐ OTHER: _____
  _____
  _____

TEXTURE METER
- RUNNY
- SOFT
- SEMI-SOFT
- SEMI-FIRM
- FIRM
- HARD

NOTES
_____
_____
_____
_____
_____
_____

RATING
☆ ☆ ☆ ☆ ☆

NAME OF CHEESE _____

FACTORY _____

RIND
- [ ] BLOOMY
- [ ] WASHED
- [ ] NATURAL
- [ ] DRY
- [ ] WHITE
- [ ] SALTY
- [ ] THICK
- [ ] SOFT
- [ ] HARD
- [ ] FUZZY
- [ ] GRITTY

ORIGIN _____

DATE _____

PRICE _____

FLAVORS
- [ ] SALTY
- [ ] GRASSY
- [ ] SWEET
- [ ] ROBUST
- [ ] CRYSTALLINE
- [ ] HERBAL
- [ ] CRUMBLY
- [ ] SKINKY
- [ ] SHARP/TANGY
- [ ] CARAMEL
- [ ] MILKY/LACTIC
- [ ] MOLDY/BLUE
- [ ] LEMON
- [ ] NUTTY
- [ ] BUTTERY/CREAMY
- [ ] EARTHY

MILK
- [ ] COW
- [ ] SHEEP
- [ ] GOAT
- [ ] RAW
- [ ] OTHER: _____

TEXTURE METER
- RUNNY
- SOFT
- SEMI-SOFT
- SEMI-FIRM
- FIRM
- HARD

NOTES
_____
_____
_____
_____
_____

RATING
☆ ☆ ☆ ☆ ☆

NAME OF CHEESE _____

FACTORY _____

RIND
- ☐ BLOOMY ☐ WASHED ☐ NATURAL ☐ DRY
  - ☐ WHITE   ☐ SALTY   ☐ THICK
  - ☐ SOFT   ☐ HARD
  - ☐ FUZZY   ☐ GRITTY

ORIGIN _____

DATE _____

PRICE _____

FLAVORS
- ☐ SALTY
- ☐ SWEET
- ☐ CRYSTALLINE
- ☐ CRUMBLY
- ☐ SHARP/TANGY
- ☐ MILKY/LACTIC
- ☐ LEMON
- ☐ BUTTERY/CREAMY
- ☐ GRASSY
- ☐ ROBUST
- ☐ HERBAL
- ☐ SKINKY
- ☐ CARAMEL
- ☐ MOLDY/BLUE
- ☐ NUTTY
- ☐ EARTHY

MILK
- ☐ COW
- ☐ SHEEP
- ☐ GOAT
- ☐ RAW
- ☐ OTHER: _____
  _____
  _____

TEXTURE METER
- RUNNY
- SOFT
- SEMI-SOFT
- SEMI-FIRM
- FIRM
- HARD

NOTES
_____
_____
_____
_____
_____

RATING ☆☆☆☆☆

NAME OF CHEESE _____

FACTORY _____

RIND

- [ ] BLOOMY
- [ ] WASHED
- [ ] NATURAL
- [ ] DRY
- [ ] WHITE
- [ ] SALTY
- [ ] THICK
- [ ] SOFT
- [ ] HARD
- [ ] FUZZY
- [ ] GRITTY

ORIGIN _____

DATE _____

PRICE _____

FLAVORS

- [ ] SALTY
- [ ] GRASSY
- [ ] SWEET
- [ ] ROBUST
- [ ] CRYSTALLINE
- [ ] HERBAL
- [ ] CRUMBLY
- [ ] SKINKY
- [ ] SHARP/TANGY
- [ ] CARAMEL
- [ ] MILKY/LACTIC
- [ ] MOLDY/BLUE
- [ ] LEMON
- [ ] NUTTY
- [ ] BUTTERY/CREAMY
- [ ] EARTHY

MILK

- [ ] COW
- [ ] SHEEP
- [ ] GOAT
- [ ] RAW
- [ ] OTHER: _____
  _____
  _____

TEXTURE METER

- RUNNY
- SOFT
- SEMI-SOFT
- SEMI-FIRM
- FIRM
- HARD

NOTES

_____
_____
_____
_____
_____
_____

RATING

☆☆☆☆☆

NAME OF CHEESE _____

FACTORY _____

RIND

- ☐ BLOOMY ☐ WASHED ☐ NATURAL ☐ DRY
  - ☐ WHITE ☐ SALTY ☐ THICK
  - ☐ SOFT ☐ HARD
  - ☐ FUZZY ☐ GRITTY

ORIGIN _____

DATE _____

PRICE _____

FLAVORS

- ☐ SALTY
- ☐ SWEET
- ☐ CRYSTALLINE
- ☐ CRUMBLY
- ☐ SHARP/TANGY
- ☐ MILKY/LACTIC
- ☐ LEMON
- ☐ BUTTERY/CREAMY
- ☐ GRASSY
- ☐ ROBUST
- ☐ HERBAL
- ☐ SKINKY
- ☐ CARAMEL
- ☐ MOLDY/BLUE
- ☐ NUTTY
- ☐ EARTHY

MILK

- ☐ COW
- ☐ SHEEP
- ☐ GOAT
- ☐ RAW
- ☐ OTHER: _____
  _____
  _____

TEXTURE METER

- RUNNY
- SOFT
- SEMI-SOFT
- SEMI-FIRM
- FIRM
- HARD

NOTES

_____
_____
_____
_____
_____

RATING

☆ ☆ ☆ ☆ ☆

NAME OF CHEESE _____

FACTORY _____

RIND
- ☐ BLOOMY ☐ WASHED ☐ NATURAL ☐ DRY
  - ☐ WHITE   ☐ SALTY   ☐ THICK
  - ☐ SOFT   ☐ HARD
  - ☐ FUZZY   ☐ GRITTY

ORIGIN _____

DATE _____

PRICE _____

FLAVORS
- ☐ SALTY
- ☐ SWEET
- ☐ CRYSTALLINE
- ☐ CRUMBLY
- ☐ SHARP/TANGY
- ☐ MILKY/LACTIC
- ☐ LEMON
- ☐ BUTTERY/CREAMY
- ☐ GRASSY
- ☐ ROBUST
- ☐ HERBAL
- ☐ SKINKY
- ☐ CARAMEL
- ☐ MOLDY/BLUE
- ☐ NUTTY
- ☐ EARTHY

MILK
- ☐ COW
- ☐ SHEEP
- ☐ GOAT
- ☐ RAW
- ☐ OTHER: _____
  _____
  _____

TEXTURE METER
- RUNNY
- SOFT
- SEMI-SOFT
- SEMI-FIRM
- FIRM
- HARD

NOTES
_____
_____
_____
_____
_____

RATING ☆☆☆☆☆

NAME OF CHEESE _____

FACTORY _____

RIND

- [ ] BLOOMY [ ] WASHED [ ] NATURAL [ ] DRY
  - [ ] WHITE [ ] SALTY [ ] THICK
  - [ ] SOFT   [ ] HARD
  - [ ] FUZZY   [ ] GRITTY

ORIGIN _____

DATE _____

PRICE _____

FLAVORS

- [ ] SALTY
- [ ] SWEET
- [ ] CRYSTALLINE
- [ ] CRUMBLY
- [ ] SHARP/TANGY
- [ ] MILKY/LACTIC
- [ ] LEMON
- [ ] BUTTERY/CREAMY
- [ ] GRASSY
- [ ] ROBUST
- [ ] HERBAL
- [ ] SKINKY
- [ ] CARAMEL
- [ ] MOLDY/BLUE
- [ ] NUTTY
- [ ] EARTHY

MILK

- [ ] COW
- [ ] SHEEP
- [ ] GOAT
- [ ] RAW
- [ ] OTHER: _____
  _____
  _____

TEXTURE METER

- RUNNY
- SOFT
- SEMI-SOFT
- SEMI-FIRM
- FIRM
- HARD

NOTES

_____
_____
_____
_____
_____
_____

RATING

☆ ☆ ☆ ☆ ☆

NAME OF CHEESE _____

FACTORY _____

RIND
- [ ] BLOOMY
- [ ] WASHED
- [ ] NATURAL
- [ ] DRY
  - [ ] WHITE
  - [ ] SALTY
  - [ ] THICK
  - [ ] SOFT
  - [ ] HARD
  - [ ] FUZZY
  - [ ] GRITTY

ORIGIN _____

DATE _____

PRICE _____

FLAVORS
- [ ] SALTY
- [ ] GRASSY
- [ ] SWEET
- [ ] ROBUST
- [ ] CRYSTALLINE
- [ ] HERBAL
- [ ] CRUMBLY
- [ ] SKINKY
- [ ] SHARP/TANGY
- [ ] CARAMEL
- [ ] MILKY/LACTIC
- [ ] MOLDY/BLUE
- [ ] LEMON
- [ ] NUTTY
- [ ] BUTTERY/CREAMY
- [ ] EARTHY

MILK
- [ ] COW
- [ ] SHEEP
- [ ] GOAT
- [ ] RAW
- [ ] OTHER: _____
  _____
  _____

TEXTURE METER
- RUNNY
- SOFT
- SEMI-SOFT
- SEMI-FIRM
- FIRM
- HARD

NOTES
_____
_____
_____
_____
_____

RATING
☆ ☆ ☆ ☆ ☆

NAME OF CHEESE _____

FACTORY _____

RIND
- ☐ BLOOMY ☐ WASHED ☐ NATURAL ☐ DRY
  - ☐ WHITE   ☐ SALTY   ☐ THICK
  - ☐ SOFT   ☐ HARD
  - ☐ FUZZY   ☐ GRITTY

ORIGIN _____

DATE _____

PRICE _____

FLAVORS
- ☐ SALTY
- ☐ SWEET
- ☐ CRYSTALLINE
- ☐ CRUMBLY
- ☐ SHARP/TANGY
- ☐ MILKY/LACTIC
- ☐ LEMON
- ☐ BUTTERY/CREAMY
- ☐ GRASSY
- ☐ ROBUST
- ☐ HERBAL
- ☐ SKINKY
- ☐ CARAMEL
- ☐ MOLDY/BLUE
- ☐ NUTTY
- ☐ EARTHY

MILK
- ☐ COW
- ☐ SHEEP
- ☐ GOAT
- ☐ RAW
- ☐ OTHER: _____
  _____
  _____

TEXTURE METER
- RUNNY
- SOFT
- SEMI-SOFT
- SEMI-FIRM
- FIRM
- HARD

NOTES
_____
_____
_____
_____
_____

RATING ☆☆☆☆☆

NAME OF CHEESE _____

FACTORY _____

RIND
- [ ] BLOOMY
- [ ] WASHED
- [ ] NATURAL
- [ ] DRY
  - [ ] WHITE
  - [ ] SALTY
  - [ ] THICK
  - [ ] SOFT
  - [ ] HARD
  - [ ] FUZZY
  - [ ] GRITTY

ORIGIN _____

DATE _____

PRICE _____

FLAVORS
- [ ] SALTY
- [ ] SWEET
- [ ] CRYSTALLINE
- [ ] CRUMBLY
- [ ] SHARP/TANGY
- [ ] MILKY/LACTIC
- [ ] LEMON
- [ ] BUTTERY/CREAMY
- [ ] GRASSY
- [ ] ROBUST
- [ ] HERBAL
- [ ] SKINKY
- [ ] CARAMEL
- [ ] MOLDY/BLUE
- [ ] NUTTY
- [ ] EARTHY

MILK
- [ ] COW
- [ ] SHEEP
- [ ] GOAT
- [ ] RAW
- [ ] OTHER: _____

TEXTURE METER
- RUNNY
- SOFT
- SEMI-SOFT
- SEMI-FIRM
- FIRM
- HARD

NOTES
_____
_____
_____
_____
_____
_____

RATING
☆ ☆ ☆ ☆ ☆

NAME OF CHEESE _____

FACTORY _____

RIND
- ☐ BLOOMY ☐ WASHED ☐ NATURAL ☐ DRY
  - ☐ WHITE   ☐ SALTY   ☐ THICK
  - ☐ SOFT   ☐ HARD
  - ☐ FUZZY   ☐ GRITTY

ORIGIN _____

DATE _____

PRICE _____

FLAVORS
- ☐ SALTY
- ☐ SWEET
- ☐ CRYSTALLINE
- ☐ CRUMBLY
- ☐ SHARP/TANGY
- ☐ MILKY/LACTIC
- ☐ LEMON
- ☐ BUTTERY/CREAMY
- ☐ GRASSY
- ☐ ROBUST
- ☐ HERBAL
- ☐ SKINKY
- ☐ CARAMEL
- ☐ MOLDY/BLUE
- ☐ NUTTY
- ☐ EARTHY

MILK
- ☐ COW
- ☐ SHEEP
- ☐ GOAT
- ☐ RAW
- ☐ OTHER: _____
  _____
  _____

TEXTURE METER
- RUNNY
- SOFT
- SEMI-SOFT
- SEMI-FIRM
- FIRM
- HARD

NOTES
_____
_____
_____
_____
_____
_____

RATING
☆ ☆ ☆ ☆ ☆

NAME OF CHEESE _____

FACTORY _____

RIND
- [ ] BLOOMY
- [ ] WASHED
- [ ] NATURAL
- [ ] DRY
  - [ ] WHITE
  - [ ] SALTY
  - [ ] THICK
  - [ ] SOFT
  - [ ] HARD
  - [ ] FUZZY
  - [ ] GRITTY

ORIGIN _____

DATE _____

PRICE _____

FLAVORS
- [ ] SALTY
- [ ] GRASSY
- [ ] SWEET
- [ ] ROBUST
- [ ] CRYSTALLINE
- [ ] HERBAL
- [ ] CRUMBLY
- [ ] SKINKY
- [ ] SHARP/TANGY
- [ ] CARAMEL
- [ ] MILKY/LACTIC
- [ ] MOLDY/BLUE
- [ ] LEMON
- [ ] NUTTY
- [ ] BUTTERY/CREAMY
- [ ] EARTHY

MILK
- [ ] COW
- [ ] SHEEP
- [ ] GOAT
- [ ] RAW
- [ ] OTHER: _____
  _____
  _____

TEXTURE METER
- RUNNY
- SOFT
- SEMI-SOFT
- SEMI-FIRM
- FIRM
- HARD

NOTES
_____
_____
_____
_____
_____
_____

RATING ☆☆☆☆☆

NAME OF CHEESE _____

FACTORY _____

RIND

- ☐ BLOOMY ☐ WASHED ☐ NATURAL ☐ DRY
  - ☐ WHITE   ☐ SALTY   ☐ THICK
  - ☐ SOFT   ☐ HARD
  - ☐ FUZZY   ☐ GRITTY

ORIGIN _____

DATE _____

PRICE _____

FLAVORS

- ☐ SALTY
- ☐ SWEET
- ☐ CRYSTALLINE
- ☐ CRUMBLY
- ☐ SHARP/TANGY
- ☐ MILKY/LACTIC
- ☐ LEMON
- ☐ BUTTERY/CREAMY
- ☐ GRASSY
- ☐ ROBUST
- ☐ HERBAL
- ☐ SKINKY
- ☐ CARAMEL
- ☐ MOLDY/BLUE
- ☐ NUTTY
- ☐ EARTHY

MILK

- ☐ COW
- ☐ SHEEP
- ☐ GOAT
- ☐ RAW
- ☐ OTHER: _____
  _____
  _____

TEXTURE METER

- RUNNY
- SOFT
- SEMI-SOFT
- SEMI-FIRM
- FIRM
- HARD

NOTES

_____
_____
_____
_____
_____

RATING

☆ ☆ ☆ ☆ ☆

NAME OF CHEESE _____

FACTORY _____

RIND
- ☐ BLOOMY ☐ WASHED ☐ NATURAL ☐ DRY
  - ☐ WHITE ☐ SALTY ☐ THICK
  - ☐ SOFT   ☐ HARD
  - ☐ FUZZY   ☐ GRITTY

ORIGIN _____

DATE _____

PRICE _____

FLAVORS
- ☐ SALTY
- ☐ SWEET
- ☐ CRYSTALLINE
- ☐ CRUMBLY
- ☐ SHARP/TANGY
- ☐ MILKY/LACTIC
- ☐ LEMON
- ☐ BUTTERY/CREAMY
- ☐ GRASSY
- ☐ ROBUST
- ☐ HERBAL
- ☐ SKINKY
- ☐ CARAMEL
- ☐ MOLDY/BLUE
- ☐ NUTTY
- ☐ EARTHY

MILK
- ☐ COW
- ☐ SHEEP
- ☐ GOAT
- ☐ RAW
- ☐ OTHER: _____

TEXTURE METER
- RUNNY
- SOFT
- SEMI-SOFT
- SEMI-FIRM
- FIRM
- HARD

NOTES
_____
_____
_____
_____
_____

RATING
☆ ☆ ☆ ☆ ☆

NAME OF CHEESE _____

FACTORY _____

RIND
☐ BLOOMY ☐ WASHED ☐ NATURAL ☐ DRY
☐ WHITE   ☐ SALTY   ☐ THICK
☐ SOFT   ☐ HARD
☐ FUZZY   ☐ GRITTY

ORIGIN _____

DATE _____

PRICE _____

FLAVORS		MILK	TEXTURE METER
☐ SALTY	☐ GRASSY	☐ COW	RUNNY
☐ SWEET	☐ ROBUST	☐ SHEEP	SOFT
☐ CRYSTALLINE	☐ HERBAL	☐ GOAT	SEMI-SOFT
☐ CRUMBLY	☐ SKINKY	☐ RAW	SEMI-FIRM
☐ SHARP/TANGY	☐ CARAMEL	☐ OTHER:	FIRM
☐ MILKY/LACTIC	☐ MOLDY/BLUE	_____	HARD
☐ LEMON	☐ NUTTY	_____	
☐ BUTTERY/CREAMY	☐ EARTHY	_____	

NOTES
_____
_____
_____
_____
_____

RATING
☆ ☆ ☆ ☆ ☆

NAME OF CHEESE _____

FACTORY _____

RIND

- ☐ BLOOMY ☐ WASHED ☐ NATURAL ☐ DRY
  - ☐ WHITE   ☐ SALTY   ☐ THICK
  - ☐ SOFT   ☐ HARD
  - ☐ FUZZY   ☐ GRITTY

ORIGIN _____

DATE _____

PRICE _____

FLAVORS

- ☐ SALTY
- ☐ SWEET
- ☐ CRYSTALLINE
- ☐ CRUMBLY
- ☐ SHARP/TANGY
- ☐ MILKY/LACTIC
- ☐ LEMON
- ☐ BUTTERY/CREAMY
- ☐ GRASSY
- ☐ ROBUST
- ☐ HERBAL
- ☐ SKINKY
- ☐ CARAMEL
- ☐ MOLDY/BLUE
- ☐ NUTTY
- ☐ EARTHY

MILK

- ☐ COW
- ☐ SHEEP
- ☐ GOAT
- ☐ RAW
- ☐ OTHER: _____
  _____
  _____

TEXTURE METER

- RUNNY
- SOFT
- SEMI-SOFT
- SEMI-FIRM
- FIRM
- HARD

NOTES

_____
_____
_____
_____
_____

RATING

☆☆☆☆☆

NAME OF CHEESE _____

FACTORY _____

RIND
- ☐ BLOOMY ☐ WASHED ☐ NATURAL ☐ DRY
  - ☐ WHITE ☐ SALTY ☐ THICK
  - ☐ SOFT ☐ HARD
  - ☐ FUZZY ☐ GRITTY

ORIGIN _____

DATE _____

PRICE _____

FLAVORS
- ☐ SALTY
- ☐ SWEET
- ☐ CRYSTALLINE
- ☐ CRUMBLY
- ☐ SHARP/TANGY
- ☐ MILKY/LACTIC
- ☐ LEMON
- ☐ BUTTERY/CREAMY
- ☐ GRASSY
- ☐ ROBUST
- ☐ HERBAL
- ☐ SKINKY
- ☐ CARAMEL
- ☐ MOLDY/BLUE
- ☐ NUTTY
- ☐ EARTHY

MILK
- ☐ COW
- ☐ SHEEP
- ☐ GOAT
- ☐ RAW
- ☐ OTHER: _____
  _____
  _____

TEXTURE METER
- RUNNY
- SOFT
- SEMI-SOFT
- SEMI-FIRM
- FIRM
- HARD

NOTES
_____
_____
_____
_____
_____

RATING ☆ ☆ ☆ ☆ ☆

NAME OF CHEESE _____

FACTORY _____

RIND

- [ ] BLOOMY [ ] WASHED [ ] NATURAL [ ] DRY
  - [ ] WHITE [ ] SALTY [ ] THICK
  - [ ] SOFT   [ ] HARD
  - [ ] FUZZY   [ ] GRITTY

ORIGIN _____

DATE _____

PRICE _____

FLAVORS

- [ ] SALTY
- [ ] SWEET
- [ ] CRYSTALLINE
- [ ] CRUMBLY
- [ ] SHARP/TANGY
- [ ] MILKY/LACTIC
- [ ] LEMON
- [ ] BUTTERY/CREAMY
- [ ] GRASSY
- [ ] ROBUST
- [ ] HERBAL
- [ ] SKINKY
- [ ] CARAMEL
- [ ] MOLDY/BLUE
- [ ] NUTTY
- [ ] EARTHY

MILK

- [ ] COW
- [ ] SHEEP
- [ ] GOAT
- [ ] RAW
- [ ] OTHER: _____

TEXTURE METER

- RUNNY
- SOFT
- SEMI-SOFT
- SEMI-FIRM
- FIRM
- HARD

NOTES

_____
_____
_____
_____
_____

RATING

☆ ☆ ☆ ☆ ☆

NAME OF CHEESE _____

FACTORY _____

RIND
- ☐ BLOOMY ☐ WASHED ☐ NATURAL ☐ DRY
  - ☐ WHITE ☐ SALTY ☐ THICK
  - ☐ SOFT   ☐ HARD
  - ☐ FUZZY   ☐ GRITTY

ORIGIN _____

DATE _____

PRICE _____

FLAVORS
- ☐ SALTY
- ☐ SWEET
- ☐ CRYSTALLINE
- ☐ CRUMBLY
- ☐ SHARP/TANGY
- ☐ MILKY/LACTIC
- ☐ LEMON
- ☐ BUTTERY/CREAMY
- ☐ GRASSY
- ☐ ROBUST
- ☐ HERBAL
- ☐ SKINKY
- ☐ CARAMEL
- ☐ MOLDY/BLUE
- ☐ NUTTY
- ☐ EARTHY

MILK
- ☐ COW
- ☐ SHEEP
- ☐ GOAT
- ☐ RAW
- ☐ OTHER: _____
  _____
  _____

TEXTURE METER
- RUNNY
- SOFT
- SEMI-SOFT
- SEMI-FIRM
- FIRM
- HARD

NOTES
_____
_____
_____
_____
_____
_____

RATING
☆ ☆ ☆ ☆ ☆

NAME OF CHEESE _____

FACTORY _____

RIND
- ☐ BLOOMY ☐ WASHED ☐ NATURAL ☐ DRY
  - ☐ WHITE ☐ SALTY ☐ THICK
  - ☐ SOFT ☐ HARD
  - ☐ FUZZY ☐ GRITTY

ORIGIN _____

DATE _____

PRICE _____

FLAVORS
- ☐ SALTY ☐ GRASSY
- ☐ SWEET ☐ ROBUST
- ☐ CRYSTALLINE ☐ HERBAL
- ☐ CRUMBLY ☐ SKINKY
- ☐ SHARP/TANGY ☐ CARAMEL
- ☐ MILKY/LACTIC ☐ MOLDY/BLUE
- ☐ LEMON ☐ NUTTY
- ☐ BUTTERY/CREAMY ☐ EARTHY

MILK
- ☐ COW
- ☐ SHEEP
- ☐ GOAT
- ☐ RAW
- ☐ OTHER: _____
  _____
  _____

TEXTURE METER
- RUNNY
- SOFT
- SEMI-SOFT
- SEMI-FIRM
- FIRM
- HARD

NOTES
_____
_____
_____
_____
_____

RATING
☆ ☆ ☆ ☆ ☆

NAME OF CHEESE _____

FACTORY _____

RIND
- ☐ BLOOMY ☐ WASHED ☐ NATURAL ☐ DRY
  - ☐ WHITE ☐ SALTY ☐ THICK
  - ☐ SOFT ☐ HARD
  - ☐ FUZZY ☐ GRITTY

ORIGIN _____

DATE _____

PRICE _____

FLAVORS
- ☐ SALTY ☐ GRASSY
- ☐ SWEET ☐ ROBUST
- ☐ CRYSTALLINE ☐ HERBAL
- ☐ CRUMBLY ☐ SKINKY
- ☐ SHARP/TANGY ☐ CARAMEL
- ☐ MILKY/LACTIC ☐ MOLDY/BLUE
- ☐ LEMON ☐ NUTTY
- ☐ BUTTERY/CREAMY ☐ EARTHY

MILK
- ☐ COW
- ☐ SHEEP
- ☐ GOAT
- ☐ RAW
- ☐ OTHER: _____
  _____
  _____

TEXTURE METER
- RUNNY
- SOFT
- SEMI-SOFT
- SEMI-FIRM
- FIRM
- HARD

NOTES
_____
_____
_____
_____
_____
_____

RATING
☆ ☆ ☆ ☆ ☆

NAME OF CHEESE _____

FACTORY _____

RIND

- [ ] BLOOMY
- [ ] WASHED
- [ ] NATURAL
- [ ] DRY
  - [ ] WHITE
  - [ ] SALTY
  - [ ] THICK
  - [ ] SOFT
  - [ ] HARD
  - [ ] FUZZY
  - [ ] GRITTY

ORIGIN _____

DATE _____

PRICE _____

FLAVORS

- [ ] SALTY
- [ ] GRASSY
- [ ] SWEET
- [ ] ROBUST
- [ ] CRYSTALLINE
- [ ] HERBAL
- [ ] CRUMBLY
- [ ] SKINKY
- [ ] SHARP/TANGY
- [ ] CARAMEL
- [ ] MILKY/LACTIC
- [ ] MOLDY/BLUE
- [ ] LEMON
- [ ] NUTTY
- [ ] BUTTERY/CREAMY
- [ ] EARTHY

MILK

- [ ] COW
- [ ] SHEEP
- [ ] GOAT
- [ ] RAW
- [ ] OTHER: _____
  _____
  _____

TEXTURE METER

- RUNNY
- SOFT
- SEMI-SOFT
- SEMI-FIRM
- FIRM
- HARD

NOTES

_____
_____
_____
_____
_____

RATING

☆ ☆ ☆ ☆ ☆

NAME OF CHEESE _____

FACTORY _____

RIND
- ☐ BLOOMY ☐ WASHED ☐ NATURAL ☐ DRY
  - ☐ WHITE   ☐ SALTY   ☐ THICK
  - ☐ SOFT   ☐ HARD
  - ☐ FUZZY   ☐ GRITTY

ORIGIN _____

DATE _____

PRICE _____

FLAVORS
- ☐ SALTY   ☐ GRASSY
- ☐ SWEET   ☐ ROBUST
- ☐ CRYSTALLINE   ☐ HERBAL
- ☐ CRUMBLY   ☐ SKINKY
- ☐ SHARP/TANGY   ☐ CARAMEL
- ☐ MILKY/LACTIC   ☐ MOLDY/BLUE
- ☐ LEMON   ☐ NUTTY
- ☐ BUTTERY/CREAMY   ☐ EARTHY

MILK
- ☐ COW
- ☐ SHEEP
- ☐ GOAT
- ☐ RAW
- ☐ OTHER: _____
  _____
  _____

TEXTURE METER
- RUNNY
- SOFT
- SEMI-SOFT
- SEMI-FIRM
- FIRM
- HARD

NOTES
_____
_____
_____
_____
_____

RATING
☆ ☆ ☆ ☆ ☆

NAME OF CHEESE _____

FACTORY _____

RIND

- ☐ BLOOMY ☐ WASHED ☐ NATURAL ☐ DRY
  - ☐ WHITE   ☐ SALTY   ☐ THICK
  - ☐ SOFT   ☐ HARD
  - ☐ FUZZY   ☐ GRITTY

ORIGIN _____

DATE _____

PRICE _____

FLAVORS

- ☐ SALTY   ☐ GRASSY
- ☐ SWEET   ☐ ROBUST
- ☐ CRYSTALLINE   ☐ HERBAL
- ☐ CRUMBLY   ☐ SKINKY
- ☐ SHARP/TANGY   ☐ CARAMEL
- ☐ MILKY/LACTIC   ☐ MOLDY/BLUE
- ☐ LEMON   ☐ NUTTY
- ☐ BUTTERY/CREAMY   ☐ EARTHY

MILK

- ☐ COW
- ☐ SHEEP
- ☐ GOAT
- ☐ RAW
- ☐ OTHER: _____
  _____
  _____

TEXTURE METER

- RUNNY
- SOFT
- SEMI-SOFT
- SEMI-FIRM
- FIRM
- HARD

NOTES

_____
_____
_____
_____
_____

RATING

☆ ☆ ☆ ☆ ☆

NAME OF CHEESE _____

FACTORY _____

RIND
- ☐ BLOOMY ☐ WASHED ☐ NATURAL ☐ DRY
  - ☐ WHITE   ☐ SALTY   ☐ THICK
  - ☐ SOFT   ☐ HARD
  - ☐ FUZZY   ☐ GRITTY

ORIGIN _____

DATE _____

PRICE _____

FLAVORS
- ☐ SALTY
- ☐ SWEET
- ☐ CRYSTALLINE
- ☐ CRUMBLY
- ☐ SHARP/TANGY
- ☐ MILKY/LACTIC
- ☐ LEMON
- ☐ BUTTERY/CREAMY
- ☐ GRASSY
- ☐ ROBUST
- ☐ HERBAL
- ☐ SKINKY
- ☐ CARAMEL
- ☐ MOLDY/BLUE
- ☐ NUTTY
- ☐ EARTHY

MILK
- ☐ COW
- ☐ SHEEP
- ☐ GOAT
- ☐ RAW
- ☐ OTHER: _____
  _____
  _____

TEXTURE METER
- RUNNY
- SOFT
- SEMI-SOFT
- SEMI-FIRM
- FIRM
- HARD

NOTES
_____
_____
_____
_____
_____

RATING ☆☆☆☆☆

NAME OF CHEESE _____

FACTORY _____

RIND
- [ ] BLOOMY [ ] WASHED [ ] NATURAL [ ] DRY
  - [ ] WHITE [ ] SALTY [ ] THICK
  - [ ] SOFT [ ] HARD
  - [ ] FUZZY [ ] GRITTY

ORIGIN _____

DATE _____

PRICE _____

FLAVORS
- [ ] SALTY
- [ ] SWEET
- [ ] CRYSTALLINE
- [ ] CRUMBLY
- [ ] SHARP/TANGY
- [ ] MILKY/LACTIC
- [ ] LEMON
- [ ] BUTTERY/CREAMY
- [ ] GRASSY
- [ ] ROBUST
- [ ] HERBAL
- [ ] SKINKY
- [ ] CARAMEL
- [ ] MOLDY/BLUE
- [ ] NUTTY
- [ ] EARTHY

MILK
- [ ] COW
- [ ] SHEEP
- [ ] GOAT
- [ ] RAW
- [ ] OTHER: _____
  _____
  _____

TEXTURE METER
- RUNNY
- SOFT
- SEMI-SOFT
- SEMI-FIRM
- FIRM
- HARD

NOTES
_____
_____
_____
_____
_____
_____

RATING
☆ ☆ ☆ ☆ ☆

NAME OF CHEESE _____

FACTORY _____

RIND

- ☐ BLOOMY   ☐ WASHED   ☐ NATURAL   ☐ DRY
  - ☐ WHITE   ☐ SALTY   ☐ THICK
  - ☐ SOFT   ☐ HARD
  - ☐ FUZZY   ☐ GRITTY

ORIGIN _____

DATE _____

PRICE _____

FLAVORS

- ☐ SALTY   ☐ GRASSY
- ☐ SWEET   ☐ ROBUST
- ☐ CRYSTALLINE   ☐ HERBAL
- ☐ CRUMBLY   ☐ SKINKY
- ☐ SHARP/TANGY   ☐ CARAMEL
- ☐ MILKY/LACTIC   ☐ MOLDY/BLUE
- ☐ LEMON   ☐ NUTTY
- ☐ BUTTERY/CREAMY ☐ EARTHY

MILK

- ☐ COW
- ☐ SHEEP
- ☐ GOAT
- ☐ RAW
- ☐ OTHER: _____
  _____
  _____

TEXTURE METER

- RUNNY
- SOFT
- SEMI-SOFT
- SEMI-FIRM
- FIRM
- HARD

NOTES

_____
_____
_____
_____
_____
_____

RATING
☆ ☆ ☆ ☆ ☆

NAME OF CHEESE _____

FACTORY _____

RIND
☐ BLOOMY ☐ WASHED ☐ NATURAL ☐ DRY
☐ WHITE ☐ SALTY ☐ THICK
☐ SOFT ☐ HARD
☐ FUZZY ☐ GRITTY

ORIGIN _____

DATE _____

PRICE _____

FLAVORS		MILK	TEXTURE METER
☐ SALTY	☐ GRASSY	☐ COW	RUNNY
☐ SWEET	☐ ROBUST	☐ SHEEP	SOFT
☐ CRYSTALLINE	☐ HERBAL	☐ GOAT	SEMI-SOFT
☐ CRUMBLY	☐ SKINKY	☐ RAW	SEMI-FIRM
☐ SHARP/TANGY	☐ CARAMEL	☐ OTHER:	FIRM
☐ MILKY/LACTIC	☐ MOLDY/BLUE	_____	HARD
☐ LEMON	☐ NUTTY	_____	
☐ BUTTERY/CREAMY	☐ EARTHY	_____	

NOTES

_____

_____

_____

_____

_____

RATING
☆ ☆ ☆ ☆ ☆

NAME OF CHEESE _____

FACTORY _____

RIND

- ☐ BLOOMY   ☐ WASHED   ☐ NATURAL   ☐ DRY
  - ☐ WHITE   ☐ SALTY   ☐ THICK
  - ☐ SOFT   ☐ HARD
  - ☐ FUZZY   ☐ GRITTY

ORIGIN _____

DATE _____

PRICE _____

FLAVORS

- ☐ SALTY   ☐ GRASSY
- ☐ SWEET   ☐ ROBUST
- ☐ CRYSTALLINE   ☐ HERBAL
- ☐ CRUMBLY   ☐ SKINKY
- ☐ SHARP/TANGY   ☐ CARAMEL
- ☐ MILKY/LACTIC   ☐ MOLDY/BLUE
- ☐ LEMON   ☐ NUTTY
- ☐ BUTTERY/CREAMY   ☐ EARTHY

MILK

- ☐ COW
- ☐ SHEEP
- ☐ GOAT
- ☐ RAW
- ☐ OTHER: _____
  _____
  _____

TEXTURE METER

- RUNNY
- SOFT
- SEMI-SOFT
- SEMI-FIRM
- FIRM
- HARD

NOTES

_____
_____
_____
_____
_____

RATING

☆ ☆ ☆ ☆ ☆

NAME OF CHEESE _____

FACTORY _____

RIND	
☐ BLOOMY ☐ WASHED ☐ NATURAL ☐ DRY	
☐ WHITE ☐ SALTY ☐ THICK	
☐ SOFT ☐ HARD	
☐ FUZZY ☐ GRITTY	

ORIGIN _____

DATE _____

PRICE _____

FLAVORS		MILK	TEXTURE METER
☐ SALTY	☐ GRASSY	☐ COW	RUNNY
☐ SWEET	☐ ROBUST	☐ SHEEP	SOFT
☐ CRYSTALLINE	☐ HERBAL	☐ GOAT	SEMI-SOFT
☐ CRUMBLY	☐ SKINKY	☐ RAW	SEMI-FIRM
☐ SHARP/TANGY	☐ CARAMEL	☐ OTHER:	FIRM
☐ MILKY/LACTIC	☐ MOLDY/BLUE	_____	HARD
☐ LEMON	☐ NUTTY	_____	
☐ BUTTERY/CREAMY	☐ EARTHY	_____	

NOTES

_____

_____

_____

_____

_____

_____

RATING
☆ ☆ ☆ ☆ ☆

NAME OF CHEESE _____

FACTORY _____

RIND

- ☐ BLOOMY ☐ WASHED ☐ NATURAL ☐ DRY
  - ☐ WHITE   ☐ SALTY   ☐ THICK
  - ☐ SOFT   ☐ HARD
  - ☐ FUZZY   ☐ GRITTY

ORIGIN _____

DATE _____

PRICE _____

FLAVORS

- ☐ SALTY
- ☐ SWEET
- ☐ CRYSTALLINE
- ☐ CRUMBLY
- ☐ SHARP/TANGY
- ☐ MILKY/LACTIC
- ☐ LEMON
- ☐ BUTTERY/CREAMY
- ☐ GRASSY
- ☐ ROBUST
- ☐ HERBAL
- ☐ SKINKY
- ☐ CARAMEL
- ☐ MOLDY/BLUE
- ☐ NUTTY
- ☐ EARTHY

MILK

- ☐ COW
- ☐ SHEEP
- ☐ GOAT
- ☐ RAW
- ☐ OTHER: _____
  _____
  _____

TEXTURE METER

- RUNNY
- SOFT
- SEMI-SOFT
- SEMI-FIRM
- FIRM
- HARD

NOTES

_____
_____
_____
_____
_____
_____

RATING

☆☆☆☆☆

NAME OF CHEESE _____

FACTORY _____

RIND
- [ ] BLOOMY
- [ ] WASHED
- [ ] NATURAL
- [ ] DRY
  - [ ] WHITE
  - [ ] SALTY
  - [ ] THICK
  - [ ] SOFT
  - [ ] HARD
  - [ ] FUZZY
  - [ ] GRITTY

ORIGIN _____

DATE _____

PRICE _____

FLAVORS
- [ ] SALTY
- [ ] GRASSY
- [ ] SWEET
- [ ] ROBUST
- [ ] CRYSTALLINE
- [ ] HERBAL
- [ ] CRUMBLY
- [ ] SKINKY
- [ ] SHARP/TANGY
- [ ] CARAMEL
- [ ] MILKY/LACTIC
- [ ] MOLDY/BLUE
- [ ] LEMON
- [ ] NUTTY
- [ ] BUTTERY/CREAMY
- [ ] EARTHY

MILK
- [ ] COW
- [ ] SHEEP
- [ ] GOAT
- [ ] RAW
- [ ] OTHER: _____
  _____
  _____

TEXTURE METER
- RUNNY
- SOFT
- SEMI-SOFT
- SEMI-FIRM
- FIRM
- HARD

NOTES
_____
_____
_____
_____
_____
_____

RATING
☆ ☆ ☆ ☆ ☆

NAME OF CHEESE _____

FACTORY _____

RIND

- ☐ BLOOMY   ☐ WASHED   ☐ NATURAL   ☐ DRY
  - ☐ WHITE   ☐ SALTY   ☐ THICK
  - ☐ SOFT   ☐ HARD
  - ☐ FUZZY   ☐ GRITTY

ORIGIN _____

DATE _____

PRICE _____

FLAVORS

- ☐ SALTY
- ☐ SWEET
- ☐ CRYSTALLINE
- ☐ CRUMBLY
- ☐ SHARP/TANGY
- ☐ MILKY/LACTIC
- ☐ LEMON
- ☐ BUTTERY/CREAMY
- ☐ GRASSY
- ☐ ROBUST
- ☐ HERBAL
- ☐ SKINKY
- ☐ CARAMEL
- ☐ MOLDY/BLUE
- ☐ NUTTY
- ☐ EARTHY

MILK

- ☐ COW
- ☐ SHEEP
- ☐ GOAT
- ☐ RAW
- ☐ OTHER: _____
  _____
  _____

TEXTURE METER

- RUNNY
- SOFT
- SEMI-SOFT
- SEMI-FIRM
- FIRM
- HARD

NOTES

_____
_____
_____
_____
_____

RATING
☆ ☆ ☆ ☆ ☆

NAME OF CHEESE _____

FACTORY _____

RIND
- ☐ BLOOMY ☐ WASHED ☐ NATURAL ☐ DRY
  - ☐ WHITE ☐ SALTY ☐ THICK
  - ☐ SOFT ☐ HARD
  - ☐ FUZZY ☐ GRITTY

ORIGIN _____

DATE _____

PRICE _____

FLAVORS
- ☐ SALTY ☐ GRASSY
- ☐ SWEET ☐ ROBUST
- ☐ CRYSTALLINE ☐ HERBAL
- ☐ CRUMBLY ☐ SKINKY
- ☐ SHARP/TANGY ☐ CARAMEL
- ☐ MILKY/LACTIC ☐ MOLDY/BLUE
- ☐ LEMON ☐ NUTTY
- ☐ BUTTERY/CREAMY ☐ EARTHY

MILK
- ☐ COW
- ☐ SHEEP
- ☐ GOAT
- ☐ RAW
- ☐ OTHER: _____

TEXTURE METER
- RUNNY
- SOFT
- SEMI-SOFT
- SEMI-FIRM
- FIRM
- HARD

NOTES
_____
_____
_____
_____
_____

RATING
☆ ☆ ☆ ☆ ☆

NAME OF CHEESE _____

FACTORY _____

RIND

- ☐ BLOOMY ☐ WASHED ☐ NATURAL ☐ DRY
  - ☐ WHITE   ☐ SALTY   ☐ THICK
  - ☐ SOFT   ☐ HARD
  - ☐ FUZZY   ☐ GRITTY

ORIGIN _____

DATE _____

PRICE _____

FLAVORS

- ☐ SALTY   ☐ GRASSY
- ☐ SWEET   ☐ ROBUST
- ☐ CRYSTALLINE   ☐ HERBAL
- ☐ CRUMBLY   ☐ SKINKY
- ☐ SHARP/TANGY   ☐ CARAMEL
- ☐ MILKY/LACTIC   ☐ MOLDY/BLUE
- ☐ LEMON   ☐ NUTTY
- ☐ BUTTERY/CREAMY ☐ EARTHY

MILK

- ☐ COW
- ☐ SHEEP
- ☐ GOAT
- ☐ RAW
- ☐ OTHER: _____
  _____
  _____

TEXTURE METER

- RUNNY
- SOFT
- SEMI-SOFT
- SEMI-FIRM
- FIRM
- HARD

NOTES

_____

_____

_____

_____

_____

RATING

☆ ☆ ☆ ☆ ☆

NAME OF CHEESE _____

FACTORY _____

RIND
- [ ] BLOOMY
- [ ] WASHED
- [ ] NATURAL
- [ ] DRY
- [ ] WHITE
- [ ] SALTY
- [ ] THICK
- [ ] SOFT
- [ ] HARD
- [ ] FUZZY
- [ ] GRITTY

ORIGIN _____

DATE _____

PRICE _____

FLAVORS
- [ ] SALTY
- [ ] GRASSY
- [ ] SWEET
- [ ] ROBUST
- [ ] CRYSTALLINE
- [ ] HERBAL
- [ ] CRUMBLY
- [ ] SKINKY
- [ ] SHARP/TANGY
- [ ] CARAMEL
- [ ] MILKY/LACTIC
- [ ] MOLDY/BLUE
- [ ] LEMON
- [ ] NUTTY
- [ ] BUTTERY/CREAMY
- [ ] EARTHY

MILK
- [ ] COW
- [ ] SHEEP
- [ ] GOAT
- [ ] RAW
- [ ] OTHER: _____
  _____
  _____

TEXTURE METER
- RUNNY
- SOFT
- SEMI-SOFT
- SEMI-FIRM
- FIRM
- HARD

NOTES
_____
_____
_____
_____
_____
_____

RATING ☆☆☆☆☆

NAME OF CHEESE _____

FACTORY _____

RIND
- ☐ BLOOMY ☐ WASHED ☐ NATURAL ☐ DRY
  - ☐ WHITE ☐ SALTY ☐ THICK
  - ☐ SOFT ☐ HARD
  - ☐ FUZZY ☐ GRITTY

ORIGIN _____

DATE _____

PRICE _____

FLAVORS
- ☐ SALTY ☐ GRASSY
- ☐ SWEET ☐ ROBUST
- ☐ CRYSTALLINE ☐ HERBAL
- ☐ CRUMBLY ☐ SKINKY
- ☐ SHARP/TANGY ☐ CARAMEL
- ☐ MILKY/LACTIC ☐ MOLDY/BLUE
- ☐ LEMON ☐ NUTTY
- ☐ BUTTERY/CREAMY ☐ EARTHY

MILK
- ☐ COW
- ☐ SHEEP
- ☐ GOAT
- ☐ RAW
- ☐ OTHER: _____
  _____
  _____

TEXTURE METER
- RUNNY
- SOFT
- SEMI-SOFT
- SEMI-FIRM
- FIRM
- HARD

NOTES
_____
_____
_____
_____
_____

RATING
☆☆☆☆☆

NAME OF CHEESE _____

FACTORY _____

RIND	
☐ BLOOMY ☐ WASHED ☐ NATURAL ☐ DRY	
☐ WHITE ☐ SALTY ☐ THICK	
☐ SOFT ☐ HARD	
☐ FUZZY ☐ GRITTY	

ORIGIN _____

DATE _____

PRICE _____

FLAVORS

- ☐ SALTY
- ☐ SWEET
- ☐ CRYSTALLINE
- ☐ CRUMBLY
- ☐ SHARP/TANGY
- ☐ MILKY/LACTIC
- ☐ LEMON
- ☐ BUTTERY/CREAMY
- ☐ GRASSY
- ☐ ROBUST
- ☐ HERBAL
- ☐ SKINKY
- ☐ CARAMEL
- ☐ MOLDY/BLUE
- ☐ NUTTY
- ☐ EARTHY

MILK

- ☐ COW
- ☐ SHEEP
- ☐ GOAT
- ☐ RAW
- ☐ OTHER: _____

TEXTURE METER

- RUNNY
- SOFT
- SEMI-SOFT
- SEMI-FIRM
- FIRM
- HARD

NOTES

_____
_____
_____
_____
_____
_____

RATING ☆☆☆☆☆

NAME OF CHEESE _____

FACTORY _____

RIND

- ☐ BLOOMY ☐ WASHED ☐ NATURAL ☐ DRY
  - ☐ WHITE   ☐ SALTY   ☐ THICK
  - ☐ SOFT   ☐ HARD
  - ☐ FUZZY   ☐ GRITTY

ORIGIN _____

DATE _____

PRICE _____

FLAVORS

- ☐ SALTY   ☐ GRASSY
- ☐ SWEET   ☐ ROBUST
- ☐ CRYSTALLINE   ☐ HERBAL
- ☐ CRUMBLY   ☐ SKINKY
- ☐ SHARP/TANGY   ☐ CARAMEL
- ☐ MILKY/LACTIC   ☐ MOLDY/BLUE
- ☐ LEMON   ☐ NUTTY
- ☐ BUTTERY/CREAMY   ☐ EARTHY

MILK

- ☐ COW
- ☐ SHEEP
- ☐ GOAT
- ☐ RAW
- ☐ OTHER:
  _____
  _____
  _____

TEXTURE METER

- RUNNY
- SOFT
- SEMI-SOFT
- SEMI-FIRM
- FIRM
- HARD

NOTES

_____
_____
_____
_____
_____

RATING

☆ ☆ ☆ ☆ ☆

NAME OF CHEESE _____

FACTORY _____

RIND

- ☐ BLOOMY   ☐ WASHED   ☐ NATURAL   ☐ DRY
  - ☐ WHITE   ☐ SALTY   ☐ THICK
  - ☐ SOFT   ☐ HARD
  - ☐ FUZZY   ☐ GRITTY

ORIGIN _____

DATE _____

PRICE _____

FLAVORS

- ☐ SALTY   ☐ GRASSY
- ☐ SWEET   ☐ ROBUST
- ☐ CRYSTALLINE   ☐ HERBAL
- ☐ CRUMBLY   ☐ SKINKY
- ☐ SHARP/TANGY   ☐ CARAMEL
- ☐ MILKY/LACTIC   ☐ MOLDY/BLUE
- ☐ LEMON   ☐ NUTTY
- ☐ BUTTERY/CREAMY   ☐ EARTHY

MILK

- ☐ COW
- ☐ SHEEP
- ☐ GOAT
- ☐ RAW
- ☐ OTHER:
  _____
  _____
  _____

TEXTURE METER

- RUNNY
- SOFT
- SEMI-SOFT
- SEMI-FIRM
- FIRM
- HARD

NOTES

_____

_____

_____

_____

_____

RATING

☆ ☆ ☆ ☆ ☆

NAME OF CHEESE _____

FACTORY _____

RIND

- [ ] BLOOMY   [ ] WASHED   [ ] NATURAL   [ ] DRY
  - [ ] WHITE   [ ] SALTY   [ ] THICK
  - [ ] SOFT   [ ] HARD
  - [ ] FUZZY   [ ] GRITTY

ORIGIN _____

DATE _____

PRICE _____

FLAVORS

- [ ] SALTY   [ ] GRASSY
- [ ] SWEET   [ ] ROBUST
- [ ] CRYSTALLINE   [ ] HERBAL
- [ ] CRUMBLY   [ ] SKINKY
- [ ] SHARP/TANGY   [ ] CARAMEL
- [ ] MILKY/LACTIC   [ ] MOLDY/BLUE
- [ ] LEMON   [ ] NUTTY
- [ ] BUTTERY/CREAMY   [ ] EARTHY

MILK

- [ ] COW
- [ ] SHEEP
- [ ] GOAT
- [ ] RAW
- [ ] OTHER:
  _____
  _____
  _____

TEXTURE METER

- RUNNY
- SOFT
- SEMI-SOFT
- SEMI-FIRM
- FIRM
- HARD

NOTES

_____
_____
_____
_____
_____
_____

RATING

☆ ☆ ☆ ☆ ☆

NAME OF CHEESE _____

FACTORY _____

RIND
- [ ] BLOOMY
- [ ] WASHED
- [ ] NATURAL
- [ ] DRY
  - [ ] WHITE
  - [ ] SALTY
  - [ ] THICK
  - [ ] SOFT
  - [ ] HARD
  - [ ] FUZZY
  - [ ] GRITTY

ORIGIN _____

DATE _____

PRICE _____

FLAVORS
- [ ] SALTY
- [ ] GRASSY
- [ ] SWEET
- [ ] ROBUST
- [ ] CRYSTALLINE
- [ ] HERBAL
- [ ] CRUMBLY
- [ ] SKINKY
- [ ] SHARP/TANGY
- [ ] CARAMEL
- [ ] MILKY/LACTIC
- [ ] MOLDY/BLUE
- [ ] LEMON
- [ ] NUTTY
- [ ] BUTTERY/CREAMY
- [ ] EARTHY

MILK
- [ ] COW
- [ ] SHEEP
- [ ] GOAT
- [ ] RAW
- [ ] OTHER: _____

TEXTURE METER
- RUNNY
- SOFT
- SEMI-SOFT
- SEMI-FIRM
- FIRM
- HARD

NOTES
_____
_____
_____
_____
_____
_____

RATING
☆ ☆ ☆ ☆ ☆

NAME OF CHEESE _____

FACTORY _____

RIND
- ☐ BLOOMY ☐ WASHED ☐ NATURAL ☐ DRY
  - ☐ WHITE ☐ SALTY ☐ THICK
  - ☐ SOFT   ☐ HARD
  - ☐ FUZZY   ☐ GRITTY

ORIGIN _____

DATE _____

PRICE _____

FLAVORS
- ☐ SALTY   ☐ GRASSY
- ☐ SWEET   ☐ ROBUST
- ☐ CRYSTALLINE   ☐ HERBAL
- ☐ CRUMBLY   ☐ SKINKY
- ☐ SHARP/TANGY   ☐ CARAMEL
- ☐ MILKY/LACTIC   ☐ MOLDY/BLUE
- ☐ LEMON   ☐ NUTTY
- ☐ BUTTERY/CREAMY ☐ EARTHY

MILK
- ☐ COW
- ☐ SHEEP
- ☐ GOAT
- ☐ RAW
- ☐ OTHER: _____
  _____
  _____

TEXTURE METER
- RUNNY
- SOFT
- SEMI-SOFT
- SEMI-FIRM
- FIRM
- HARD

NOTES
_____
_____
_____
_____
_____

RATING
☆ ☆ ☆ ☆ ☆

NAME OF CHEESE _____

FACTORY _____

RIND

- [ ] BLOOMY [ ] WASHED [ ] NATURAL [ ] DRY
  - [ ] WHITE   [ ] SALTY   [ ] THICK
  - [ ] SOFT   [ ] HARD
  - [ ] FUZZY   [ ] GRITTY

ORIGIN _____

DATE _____

PRICE _____

FLAVORS

- [ ] SALTY   [ ] GRASSY
- [ ] SWEET   [ ] ROBUST
- [ ] CRYSTALLINE   [ ] HERBAL
- [ ] CRUMBLY   [ ] SKINKY
- [ ] SHARP/TANGY   [ ] CARAMEL
- [ ] MILKY/LACTIC   [ ] MOLDY/BLUE
- [ ] LEMON   [ ] NUTTY
- [ ] BUTTERY/CREAMY   [ ] EARTHY

MILK

- [ ] COW
- [ ] SHEEP
- [ ] GOAT
- [ ] RAW
- [ ] OTHER:
  _____
  _____
  _____

TEXTURE METER

- RUNNY
- SOFT
- SEMI-SOFT
- SEMI-FIRM
- FIRM
- HARD

NOTES

_____
_____
_____
_____
_____

RATING ☆☆☆☆☆

NAME OF CHEESE _____

FACTORY _____

RIND

- ☐ BLOOMY ☐ WASHED ☐ NATURAL ☐ DRY
  - ☐ WHITE ☐ SALTY ☐ THICK
  - ☐ SOFT ☐ HARD
  - ☐ FUZZY ☐ GRITTY

ORIGIN _____

DATE _____

PRICE _____

FLAVORS

- ☐ SALTY
- ☐ SWEET
- ☐ CRYSTALLINE
- ☐ CRUMBLY
- ☐ SHARP/TANGY
- ☐ MILKY/LACTIC
- ☐ LEMON
- ☐ BUTTERY/CREAMY
- ☐ GRASSY
- ☐ ROBUST
- ☐ HERBAL
- ☐ SKINKY
- ☐ CARAMEL
- ☐ MOLDY/BLUE
- ☐ NUTTY
- ☐ EARTHY

MILK

- ☐ COW
- ☐ SHEEP
- ☐ GOAT
- ☐ RAW
- ☐ OTHER: _____
  _____
  _____

TEXTURE METER

- RUNNY
- SOFT
- SEMI-SOFT
- SEMI-FIRM
- FIRM
- HARD

NOTES

_____
_____
_____
_____
_____

RATING

☆ ☆ ☆ ☆ ☆

NAME OF CHEESE _____

FACTORY _____

RIND
☐ BLOOMY ☐ WASHED ☐ NATURAL ☐ DRY
☐ WHITE ☐ SALTY ☐ THICK
☐ SOFT ☐ HARD
☐ FUZZY ☐ GRITTY

ORIGIN _____

DATE _____

PRICE _____

FLAVORS		MILK	TEXTURE METER
☐ SALTY	☐ GRASSY	☐ COW	RUNNY
☐ SWEET	☐ ROBUST	☐ SHEEP	SOFT
☐ CRYSTALLINE	☐ HERBAL	☐ GOAT	SEMI-SOFT
☐ CRUMBLY	☐ SKINKY	☐ RAW	SEMI-FIRM
☐ SHARP/TANGY	☐ CARAMEL	☐ OTHER:	FIRM
☐ MILKY/LACTIC	☐ MOLDY/BLUE	_____	HARD
☐ LEMON	☐ NUTTY	_____	
☐ BUTTERY/CREAMY	☐ EARTHY	_____	

NOTES
_____
_____
_____
_____
_____
_____

RATING
☆ ☆ ☆ ☆ ☆

NAME OF CHEESE _____

FACTORY _____

RIND
- ☐ BLOOMY ☐ WASHED ☐ NATURAL ☐ DRY
  - ☐ WHITE   ☐ SALTY   ☐ THICK
  - ☐ SOFT   ☐ HARD
  - ☐ FUZZY   ☐ GRITTY

ORIGIN _____

DATE _____

PRICE _____

FLAVORS
- ☐ SALTY
- ☐ SWEET
- ☐ CRYSTALLINE
- ☐ CRUMBLY
- ☐ SHARP/TANGY
- ☐ MILKY/LACTIC
- ☐ LEMON
- ☐ BUTTERY/CREAMY
- ☐ GRASSY
- ☐ ROBUST
- ☐ HERBAL
- ☐ SKINKY
- ☐ CARAMEL
- ☐ MOLDY/BLUE
- ☐ NUTTY
- ☐ EARTHY

MILK
- ☐ COW
- ☐ SHEEP
- ☐ GOAT
- ☐ RAW
- ☐ OTHER: _____
  _____
  _____

TEXTURE METER
- RUNNY
- SOFT
- SEMI-SOFT
- SEMI-FIRM
- FIRM
- HARD

NOTES
_____
_____
_____
_____
_____

RATING
☆ ☆ ☆ ☆ ☆

NAME OF CHEESE _____

FACTORY _____

RIND	
☐ BLOOMY ☐ WASHED	☐ NATURAL ☐ DRY
☐ WHITE ☐ SALTY	☐ THICK
☐ SOFT	☐ HARD
☐ FUZZY	☐ GRITTY

ORIGIN _____

DATE _____

PRICE _____

FLAVORS	
☐ SALTY	☐ GRASSY
☐ SWEET	☐ ROBUST
☐ CRYSTALLINE	☐ HERBAL
☐ CRUMBLY	☐ SKINKY
☐ SHARP/TANGY	☐ CARAMEL
☐ MILKY/LACTIC	☐ MOLDY/BLUE
☐ LEMON	☐ NUTTY
☐ BUTTERY/CREAMY	☐ EARTHY

MILK

☐ COW
☐ SHEEP
☐ GOAT
☐ RAW
☐ OTHER:
_____
_____
_____

TEXTURE METER

- RUNNY
- SOFT
- SEMI-SOFT
- SEMI-FIRM
- FIRM
- HARD

NOTES

_____
_____
_____
_____
_____
_____

RATING

☆ ☆ ☆ ☆ ☆

NAME OF CHEESE _____

FACTORY _____

RIND

- ☐ BLOOMY ☐ WASHED ☐ NATURAL ☐ DRY
  - ☐ WHITE ☐ SALTY ☐ THICK
  - ☐ SOFT ☐ HARD
  - ☐ FUZZY ☐ GRITTY

ORIGIN _____

DATE _____

PRICE _____

FLAVORS

- ☐ SALTY
- ☐ SWEET
- ☐ CRYSTALLINE
- ☐ CRUMBLY
- ☐ SHARP/TANGY
- ☐ MILKY/LACTIC
- ☐ LEMON
- ☐ BUTTERY/CREAMY
- ☐ GRASSY
- ☐ ROBUST
- ☐ HERBAL
- ☐ SKINKY
- ☐ CARAMEL
- ☐ MOLDY/BLUE
- ☐ NUTTY
- ☐ EARTHY

MILK

- ☐ COW
- ☐ SHEEP
- ☐ GOAT
- ☐ RAW
- ☐ OTHER: _____

TEXTURE METER

- RUNNY
- SOFT
- SEMI-SOFT
- SEMI-FIRM
- FIRM
- HARD

NOTES

_____
_____
_____
_____
_____

RATING

☆☆☆☆☆

NAME OF CHEESE _____

FACTORY _____

RIND
- ☐ BLOOMY   ☐ WASHED   ☐ NATURAL   ☐ DRY
  - ☐ WHITE   ☐ SALTY   ☐ THICK
  - ☐ SOFT   ☐ HARD
  - ☐ FUZZY   ☐ GRITTY

ORIGIN _____

DATE _____

PRICE _____

FLAVORS
- ☐ SALTY   ☐ GRASSY
- ☐ SWEET   ☐ ROBUST
- ☐ CRYSTALLINE   ☐ HERBAL
- ☐ CRUMBLY   ☐ SKINKY
- ☐ SHARP/TANGY   ☐ CARAMEL
- ☐ MILKY/LACTIC   ☐ MOLDY/BLUE
- ☐ LEMON   ☐ NUTTY
- ☐ BUTTERY/CREAMY   ☐ EARTHY

MILK
- ☐ COW
- ☐ SHEEP
- ☐ GOAT
- ☐ RAW
- ☐ OTHER: _____
  _____
  _____

TEXTURE METER
- RUNNY
- SOFT
- SEMI-SOFT
- SEMI-FIRM
- FIRM
- HARD

NOTES
_____
_____
_____
_____
_____

RATING ☆ ☆ ☆ ☆ ☆

NAME OF CHEESE _____

FACTORY _____

RIND
- ☐ BLOOMY ☐ WASHED ☐ NATURAL ☐ DRY
  - ☐ WHITE   ☐ SALTY   ☐ THICK
  - ☐ SOFT   ☐ HARD
  - ☐ FUZZY   ☐ GRITTY

ORIGIN _____

DATE _____

PRICE _____

FLAVORS
- ☐ SALTY
- ☐ SWEET
- ☐ CRYSTALLINE
- ☐ CRUMBLY
- ☐ SHARP/TANGY
- ☐ MILKY/LACTIC
- ☐ LEMON
- ☐ BUTTERY/CREAMY
- ☐ GRASSY
- ☐ ROBUST
- ☐ HERBAL
- ☐ SKINKY
- ☐ CARAMEL
- ☐ MOLDY/BLUE
- ☐ NUTTY
- ☐ EARTHY

MILK
- ☐ COW
- ☐ SHEEP
- ☐ GOAT
- ☐ RAW
- ☐ OTHER: _____
  _____
  _____

TEXTURE METER
- RUNNY
- SOFT
- SEMI-SOFT
- SEMI-FIRM
- FIRM
- HARD

NOTES
_____
_____
_____
_____
_____

RATING
☆ ☆ ☆ ☆ ☆

NAME OF CHEESE _____

FACTORY _____

RIND

- [ ] BLOOMY
- [ ] WASHED
- [ ] NATURAL
- [ ] DRY
  - [ ] WHITE
  - [ ] SALTY
  - [ ] THICK
  - [ ] SOFT
  - [ ] HARD
  - [ ] FUZZY
  - [ ] GRITTY

ORIGIN _____

DATE _____

PRICE _____

FLAVORS

- [ ] SALTY
- [ ] SWEET
- [ ] CRYSTALLINE
- [ ] CRUMBLY
- [ ] SHARP/TANGY
- [ ] MILKY/LACTIC
- [ ] LEMON
- [ ] BUTTERY/CREAMY
- [ ] GRASSY
- [ ] ROBUST
- [ ] HERBAL
- [ ] SKINKY
- [ ] CARAMEL
- [ ] MOLDY/BLUE
- [ ] NUTTY
- [ ] EARTHY

MILK

- [ ] COW
- [ ] SHEEP
- [ ] GOAT
- [ ] RAW
- [ ] OTHER: _____
  _____
  _____

TEXTURE METER

- RUNNY
- SOFT
- SEMI-SOFT
- SEMI-FIRM
- FIRM
- HARD

NOTES

_____
_____
_____
_____
_____

RATING

☆ ☆ ☆ ☆ ☆

NAME OF CHEESE _____

FACTORY _____

RIND
- [ ] BLOOMY
  - [ ] WHITE
  - [ ] SOFT
  - [ ] FUZZY
- [ ] WASHED
  - [ ] SALTY
- [ ] NATURAL
  - [ ] THICK
  - [ ] HARD
  - [ ] GRITTY
- [ ] DRY

ORIGIN _____

DATE _____

PRICE _____

FLAVORS
- [ ] SALTY
- [ ] SWEET
- [ ] CRYSTALLINE
- [ ] CRUMBLY
- [ ] SHARP/TANGY
- [ ] MILKY/LACTIC
- [ ] LEMON
- [ ] BUTTERY/CREAMY
- [ ] GRASSY
- [ ] ROBUST
- [ ] HERBAL
- [ ] SKINKY
- [ ] CARAMEL
- [ ] MOLDY/BLUE
- [ ] NUTTY
- [ ] EARTHY

MILK
- [ ] COW
- [ ] SHEEP
- [ ] GOAT
- [ ] RAW
- [ ] OTHER: _____
  _____
  _____

TEXTURE METER
- RUNNY
- SOFT
- SEMI-SOFT
- SEMI-FIRM
- FIRM
- HARD

NOTES
_____
_____
_____
_____
_____

RATING ☆☆☆☆☆

NAME OF CHEESE _____

FACTORY _____

RIND
- ☐ BLOOMY ☐ WASHED ☐ NATURAL ☐ DRY
  - ☐ WHITE   ☐ SALTY   ☐ THICK
  - ☐ SOFT   ☐ HARD
  - ☐ FUZZY   ☐ GRITTY

ORIGIN _____

DATE _____

PRICE _____

FLAVORS
- ☐ SALTY   ☐ GRASSY
- ☐ SWEET   ☐ ROBUST
- ☐ CRYSTALLINE   ☐ HERBAL
- ☐ CRUMBLY   ☐ SKINKY
- ☐ SHARP/TANGY   ☐ CARAMEL
- ☐ MILKY/LACTIC   ☐ MOLDY/BLUE
- ☐ LEMON   ☐ NUTTY
- ☐ BUTTERY/CREAMY ☐ EARTHY

MILK
- ☐ COW
- ☐ SHEEP
- ☐ GOAT
- ☐ RAW
- ☐ OTHER: _____
  _____
  _____

TEXTURE METER
- RUNNY
- SOFT
- SEMI-SOFT
- SEMI-FIRM
- FIRM
- HARD

NOTES
_____
_____
_____
_____
_____
_____

RATING
☆ ☆ ☆ ☆ ☆

NAME OF CHEESE _____

FACTORY _____

RIND
- [ ] BLOOMY
- [ ] WASHED
- [ ] NATURAL
- [ ] DRY
  - [ ] WHITE
  - [ ] SALTY
  - [ ] THICK
  - [ ] SOFT
  - [ ] HARD
  - [ ] FUZZY
  - [ ] GRITTY

ORIGIN _____

DATE _____

PRICE _____

FLAVORS
- [ ] SALTY
- [ ] GRASSY
- [ ] SWEET
- [ ] ROBUST
- [ ] CRYSTALLINE
- [ ] HERBAL
- [ ] CRUMBLY
- [ ] SKINKY
- [ ] SHARP/TANGY
- [ ] CARAMEL
- [ ] MILKY/LACTIC
- [ ] MOLDY/BLUE
- [ ] LEMON
- [ ] NUTTY
- [ ] BUTTERY/CREAMY
- [ ] EARTHY

MILK
- [ ] COW
- [ ] SHEEP
- [ ] GOAT
- [ ] RAW
- [ ] OTHER: _____
  _____
  _____

TEXTURE METER
- RUNNY
- SOFT
- SEMI-SOFT
- SEMI-FIRM
- FIRM
- HARD

NOTES
_____
_____
_____
_____
_____
_____

RATING
☆ ☆ ☆ ☆ ☆

NAME OF CHEESE _____

FACTORY _____

RIND
- [ ] BLOOMY
- [ ] WASHED
- [ ] NATURAL
- [ ] DRY
  - [ ] WHITE
  - [ ] SALTY
  - [ ] THICK
  - [ ] SOFT
  - [ ] HARD
  - [ ] FUZZY
  - [ ] GRITTY

ORIGIN _____

DATE _____

PRICE _____

FLAVORS
- [ ] SALTY
- [ ] GRASSY
- [ ] SWEET
- [ ] ROBUST
- [ ] CRYSTALLINE
- [ ] HERBAL
- [ ] CRUMBLY
- [ ] SKINKY
- [ ] SHARP/TANGY
- [ ] CARAMEL
- [ ] MILKY/LACTIC
- [ ] MOLDY/BLUE
- [ ] LEMON
- [ ] NUTTY
- [ ] BUTTERY/CREAMY
- [ ] EARTHY

MILK
- [ ] COW
- [ ] SHEEP
- [ ] GOAT
- [ ] RAW
- [ ] OTHER: _____

TEXTURE METER
- RUNNY
- SOFT
- SEMI-SOFT
- SEMI-FIRM
- FIRM
- HARD

NOTES
_____
_____
_____
_____
_____

RATING
☆ ☆ ☆ ☆ ☆

NAME OF CHEESE _____

FACTORY _____

RIND
- [ ] BLOOMY
- [ ] WASHED
- [ ] NATURAL
- [ ] DRY
  - [ ] WHITE
  - [ ] SALTY
  - [ ] THICK
  - [ ] SOFT
  - [ ] HARD
  - [ ] FUZZY
  - [ ] GRITTY

ORIGIN _____

DATE _____

PRICE _____

FLAVORS
- [ ] SALTY
- [ ] GRASSY
- [ ] SWEET
- [ ] ROBUST
- [ ] CRYSTALLINE
- [ ] HERBAL
- [ ] CRUMBLY
- [ ] SKINKY
- [ ] SHARP/TANGY
- [ ] CARAMEL
- [ ] MILKY/LACTIC
- [ ] MOLDY/BLUE
- [ ] LEMON
- [ ] NUTTY
- [ ] BUTTERY/CREAMY
- [ ] EARTHY

MILK
- [ ] COW
- [ ] SHEEP
- [ ] GOAT
- [ ] RAW
- [ ] OTHER: _____

TEXTURE METER
- RUNNY
- SOFT
- SEMI-SOFT
- SEMI-FIRM
- FIRM
- HARD

NOTES
_____
_____
_____
_____
_____
_____

RATING ☆☆☆☆☆

NAME OF CHEESE _____

FACTORY _____

RIND
- ☐ BLOOMY ☐ WASHED ☐ NATURAL ☐ DRY
  - ☐ WHITE ☐ SALTY ☐ THICK
  - ☐ SOFT ☐ HARD
  - ☐ FUZZY ☐ GRITTY

ORIGIN _____

DATE _____

PRICE _____

FLAVORS
- ☐ SALTY ☐ GRASSY
- ☐ SWEET ☐ ROBUST
- ☐ CRYSTALLINE ☐ HERBAL
- ☐ CRUMBLY ☐ SKINKY
- ☐ SHARP/TANGY ☐ CARAMEL
- ☐ MILKY/LACTIC ☐ MOLDY/BLUE
- ☐ LEMON ☐ NUTTY
- ☐ BUTTERY/CREAMY ☐ EARTHY

MILK
- ☐ COW
- ☐ SHEEP
- ☐ GOAT
- ☐ RAW
- ☐ OTHER: _____
  _____
  _____

TEXTURE METER
- RUNNY
- SOFT
- SEMI-SOFT
- SEMI-FIRM
- FIRM
- HARD

NOTES
_____
_____
_____
_____
_____
_____

RATING ☆ ☆ ☆ ☆ ☆

NAME OF CHEESE _____

FACTORY _____

RIND

- ☐ BLOOMY ☐ WASHED ☐ NATURAL ☐ DRY
  - ☐ WHITE   ☐ SALTY   ☐ THICK
  - ☐ SOFT   ☐ HARD
  - ☐ FUZZY   ☐ GRITTY

ORIGIN _____

DATE _____

PRICE _____

FLAVORS

- ☐ SALTY   ☐ GRASSY
- ☐ SWEET   ☐ ROBUST
- ☐ CRYSTALLINE   ☐ HERBAL
- ☐ CRUMBLY   ☐ SKINKY
- ☐ SHARP/TANGY   ☐ CARAMEL
- ☐ MILKY/LACTIC ☐ MOLDY/BLUE
- ☐ LEMON   ☐ NUTTY
- ☐ BUTTERY/CREAMY ☐ EARTHY

MILK

- ☐ COW
- ☐ SHEEP
- ☐ GOAT
- ☐ RAW
- ☐ OTHER: _____
  _____
  _____

TEXTURE METER

- RUNNY
- SOFT
- SEMI-SOFT
- SEMI-FIRM
- FIRM
- HARD

NOTES

_____
_____
_____
_____
_____

RATING

☆ ☆ ☆ ☆ ☆

NAME OF CHEESE _____

FACTORY _____

RIND
- ☐ BLOOMY ☐ WASHED ☐ NATURAL ☐ DRY
  - ☐ WHITE ☐ SALTY ☐ THICK
  - ☐ SOFT   ☐ HARD
  - ☐ FUZZY ☐ GRITTY

ORIGIN _____

DATE _____

PRICE _____

FLAVORS
- ☐ SALTY   ☐ GRASSY
- ☐ SWEET   ☐ ROBUST
- ☐ CRYSTALLINE   ☐ HERBAL
- ☐ CRUMBLY   ☐ SKINKY
- ☐ SHARP/TANGY   ☐ CARAMEL
- ☐ MILKY/LACTIC   ☐ MOLDY/BLUE
- ☐ LEMON   ☐ NUTTY
- ☐ BUTTERY/CREAMY ☐ EARTHY

MILK
- ☐ COW
- ☐ SHEEP
- ☐ GOAT
- ☐ RAW
- ☐ OTHER: _____
  _____
  _____

TEXTURE METER
- RUNNY
- SOFT
- SEMI-SOFT
- SEMI-FIRM
- FIRM
- HARD

NOTES
_____
_____
_____
_____
_____

RATING
☆ ☆ ☆ ☆ ☆

NAME OF CHEESE _____

FACTORY _____

RIND

- ☐ BLOOMY ☐ WASHED ☐ NATURAL ☐ DRY
  - ☐ WHITE   ☐ SALTY   ☐ THICK
  - ☐ SOFT   ☐ HARD
  - ☐ FUZZY   ☐ GRITTY

ORIGIN _____

DATE _____

PRICE _____

FLAVORS

- ☐ SALTY
- ☐ SWEET
- ☐ CRYSTALLINE
- ☐ CRUMBLY
- ☐ SHARP/TANGY
- ☐ MILKY/LACTIC
- ☐ LEMON
- ☐ BUTTERY/CREAMY
- ☐ GRASSY
- ☐ ROBUST
- ☐ HERBAL
- ☐ SKINKY
- ☐ CARAMEL
- ☐ MOLDY/BLUE
- ☐ NUTTY
- ☐ EARTHY

MILK

- ☐ COW
- ☐ SHEEP
- ☐ GOAT
- ☐ RAW
- ☐ OTHER: _____
  _____
  _____

TEXTURE METER

- RUNNY
- SOFT
- SEMI-SOFT
- SEMI-FIRM
- FIRM
- HARD

NOTES

_____
_____
_____
_____
_____
_____

RATING ☆☆☆☆☆

NAME OF CHEESE _____

FACTORY _____

RIND

- [ ] BLOOMY
- [ ] WASHED
- [ ] NATURAL
- [ ] DRY
  - [ ] WHITE
  - [ ] SALTY
  - [ ] THICK
  - [ ] SOFT
  - [ ] HARD
  - [ ] FUZZY
  - [ ] GRITTY

ORIGIN _____

DATE _____

PRICE _____

FLAVORS

- [ ] SALTY
- [ ] SWEET
- [ ] CRYSTALLINE
- [ ] CRUMBLY
- [ ] SHARP/TANGY
- [ ] MILKY/LACTIC
- [ ] LEMON
- [ ] BUTTERY/CREAMY
- [ ] GRASSY
- [ ] ROBUST
- [ ] HERBAL
- [ ] SKINKY
- [ ] CARAMEL
- [ ] MOLDY/BLUE
- [ ] NUTTY
- [ ] EARTHY

MILK

- [ ] COW
- [ ] SHEEP
- [ ] GOAT
- [ ] RAW
- [ ] OTHER: _____
  _____
  _____

TEXTURE METER

- RUNNY
- SOFT
- SEMI-SOFT
- SEMI-FIRM
- FIRM
- HARD

NOTES

_____
_____
_____
_____
_____
_____

RATING

☆ ☆ ☆ ☆ ☆

NAME OF CHEESE _____

FACTORY _____

RIND

- ☐ BLOOMY   ☐ WASHED   ☐ NATURAL   ☐ DRY
  - ☐ WHITE   ☐ SALTY   ☐ THICK
  - ☐ SOFT   ☐ HARD
  - ☐ FUZZY   ☐ GRITTY

ORIGIN _____

DATE _____

PRICE _____

FLAVORS

- ☐ SALTY
- ☐ SWEET
- ☐ CRYSTALLINE
- ☐ CRUMBLY
- ☐ SHARP/TANGY
- ☐ MILKY/LACTIC
- ☐ LEMON
- ☐ BUTTERY/CREAMY
- ☐ GRASSY
- ☐ ROBUST
- ☐ HERBAL
- ☐ SKINKY
- ☐ CARAMEL
- ☐ MOLDY/BLUE
- ☐ NUTTY
- ☐ EARTHY

MILK

- ☐ COW
- ☐ SHEEP
- ☐ GOAT
- ☐ RAW
- ☐ OTHER: _____

TEXTURE METER

- RUNNY
- SOFT
- SEMI-SOFT
- SEMI-FIRM
- FIRM
- HARD

NOTES

_____
_____
_____
_____
_____

RATING

☆ ☆ ☆ ☆ ☆

NAME OF CHEESE _____

FACTORY _____

RIND
- [ ] BLOOMY
- [ ] WASHED
- [ ] NATURAL
- [ ] DRY
  - [ ] WHITE
  - [ ] SALTY
  - [ ] THICK
  - [ ] SOFT
  - [ ] HARD
  - [ ] FUZZY
  - [ ] GRITTY

ORIGIN _____

DATE _____

PRICE _____

FLAVORS
- [ ] SALTY
- [ ] GRASSY
- [ ] SWEET
- [ ] ROBUST
- [ ] CRYSTALLINE
- [ ] HERBAL
- [ ] CRUMBLY
- [ ] SKINKY
- [ ] SHARP/TANGY
- [ ] CARAMEL
- [ ] MILKY/LACTIC
- [ ] MOLDY/BLUE
- [ ] LEMON
- [ ] NUTTY
- [ ] BUTTERY/CREAMY
- [ ] EARTHY

MILK
- [ ] COW
- [ ] SHEEP
- [ ] GOAT
- [ ] RAW
- [ ] OTHER: _____
  _____
  _____

TEXTURE METER
- RUNNY
- SOFT
- SEMI-SOFT
- SEMI-FIRM
- FIRM
- HARD

NOTES
_____
_____
_____
_____
_____

RATING ☆☆☆☆☆

NAME OF CHEESE _____

FACTORY _____

RIND

- [ ] BLOOMY
- [ ] WASHED
- [ ] NATURAL
- [ ] DRY
  - [ ] WHITE
  - [ ] SALTY
  - [ ] THICK
  - [ ] SOFT
  - [ ] HARD
  - [ ] FUZZY
  - [ ] GRITTY

ORIGIN _____

DATE _____

PRICE _____

FLAVORS

- [ ] SALTY
- [ ] SWEET
- [ ] CRYSTALLINE
- [ ] CRUMBLY
- [ ] SHARP/TANGY
- [ ] MILKY/LACTIC
- [ ] LEMON
- [ ] BUTTERY/CREAMY
- [ ] GRASSY
- [ ] ROBUST
- [ ] HERBAL
- [ ] SKINKY
- [ ] CARAMEL
- [ ] MOLDY/BLUE
- [ ] NUTTY
- [ ] EARTHY

MILK

- [ ] COW
- [ ] SHEEP
- [ ] GOAT
- [ ] RAW
- [ ] OTHER: _____
  _____
  _____

TEXTURE METER

- RUNNY
- SOFT
- SEMI-SOFT
- SEMI-FIRM
- FIRM
- HARD

NOTES

_____
_____
_____
_____
_____

RATING ☆☆☆☆☆

NAME OF CHEESE _____

FACTORY _____

RIND
- [ ] BLOOMY   [ ] WASHED   [ ] NATURAL   [ ] DRY
  - [ ] WHITE   [ ] SALTY   [ ] THICK
  - [ ] SOFT   [ ] HARD
  - [ ] FUZZY   [ ] GRITTY

ORIGIN _____

DATE _____

PRICE _____

FLAVORS
- [ ] SALTY
- [ ] SWEET
- [ ] CRYSTALLINE
- [ ] CRUMBLY
- [ ] SHARP/TANGY
- [ ] MILKY/LACTIC
- [ ] LEMON
- [ ] BUTTERY/CREAMY
- [ ] GRASSY
- [ ] ROBUST
- [ ] HERBAL
- [ ] SKINKY
- [ ] CARAMEL
- [ ] MOLDY/BLUE
- [ ] NUTTY
- [ ] EARTHY

MILK
- [ ] COW
- [ ] SHEEP
- [ ] GOAT
- [ ] RAW
- [ ] OTHER: _____
  _____
  _____

TEXTURE METER
- RUNNY
- SOFT
- SEMI-SOFT
- SEMI-FIRM
- FIRM
- HARD

NOTES
_____
_____
_____
_____
_____
_____

RATING ☆☆☆☆☆

NAME OF CHEESE _____

FACTORY _____

RIND
- ☐ BLOOMY ☐ WASHED ☐ NATURAL ☐ DRY
  - ☐ WHITE ☐ SALTY ☐ THICK
  - ☐ SOFT   ☐ HARD
  - ☐ FUZZY   ☐ GRITTY

ORIGIN _____

DATE _____

PRICE _____

FLAVORS
- ☐ SALTY
- ☐ SWEET
- ☐ CRYSTALLINE
- ☐ CRUMBLY
- ☐ SHARP/TANGY
- ☐ MILKY/LACTIC
- ☐ LEMON
- ☐ BUTTERY/CREAMY
- ☐ GRASSY
- ☐ ROBUST
- ☐ HERBAL
- ☐ SKINKY
- ☐ CARAMEL
- ☐ MOLDY/BLUE
- ☐ NUTTY
- ☐ EARTHY

MILK
- ☐ COW
- ☐ SHEEP
- ☐ GOAT
- ☐ RAW
- ☐ OTHER: _____
  _____
  _____

TEXTURE METER
- RUNNY
- SOFT
- SEMI-SOFT
- SEMI-FIRM
- FIRM
- HARD

NOTES
_____
_____
_____
_____
_____

RATING
☆ ☆ ☆ ☆ ☆

NAME OF CHEESE _____

FACTORY _____

RIND

- [ ] BLOOMY [ ] WASHED [ ] NATURAL [ ] DRY
  - [ ] WHITE [ ] SALTY [ ] THICK
  - [ ] SOFT   [ ] HARD
  - [ ] FUZZY   [ ] GRITTY

ORIGIN _____

DATE _____

PRICE _____

FLAVORS

- [ ] SALTY
- [ ] SWEET
- [ ] CRYSTALLINE
- [ ] CRUMBLY
- [ ] SHARP/TANGY
- [ ] MILKY/LACTIC
- [ ] LEMON
- [ ] BUTTERY/CREAMY
- [ ] GRASSY
- [ ] ROBUST
- [ ] HERBAL
- [ ] SKINKY
- [ ] CARAMEL
- [ ] MOLDY/BLUE
- [ ] NUTTY
- [ ] EARTHY

MILK

- [ ] COW
- [ ] SHEEP
- [ ] GOAT
- [ ] RAW
- [ ] OTHER: _____
  _____
  _____

TEXTURE METER

- RUNNY
- SOFT
- SEMI-SOFT
- SEMI-FIRM
- FIRM
- HARD

NOTES

_____
_____
_____
_____
_____

RATING

☆ ☆ ☆ ☆ ☆

NAME OF CHEESE _____

FACTORY _____

RIND
- [ ] BLOOMY
- [ ] WASHED
- [ ] NATURAL
- [ ] DRY
  - [ ] WHITE
  - [ ] SALTY
  - [ ] THICK
  - [ ] SOFT
  - [ ] HARD
  - [ ] FUZZY
  - [ ] GRITTY

ORIGIN _____

DATE _____

PRICE _____

FLAVORS
- [ ] SALTY
- [ ] SWEET
- [ ] CRYSTALLINE
- [ ] CRUMBLY
- [ ] SHARP/TANGY
- [ ] MILKY/LACTIC
- [ ] LEMON
- [ ] BUTTERY/CREAMY
- [ ] GRASSY
- [ ] ROBUST
- [ ] HERBAL
- [ ] SKINKY
- [ ] CARAMEL
- [ ] MOLDY/BLUE
- [ ] NUTTY
- [ ] EARTHY

MILK
- [ ] COW
- [ ] SHEEP
- [ ] GOAT
- [ ] RAW
- [ ] OTHER: _____
  _____
  _____

TEXTURE METER
- RUNNY
- SOFT
- SEMI-SOFT
- SEMI-FIRM
- FIRM
- HARD

NOTES
_____
_____
_____
_____
_____

RATING ☆ ☆ ☆ ☆ ☆

NAME OF CHEESE _____

FACTORY _____

RIND
- ☐ BLOOMY ☐ WASHED ☐ NATURAL ☐ DRY
  - ☐ WHITE ☐ SALTY ☐ THICK
  - ☐ SOFT   ☐ HARD
  - ☐ FUZZY   ☐ GRITTY

ORIGIN _____

DATE _____

PRICE _____

FLAVORS
- ☐ SALTY
- ☐ SWEET
- ☐ CRYSTALLINE
- ☐ CRUMBLY
- ☐ SHARP/TANGY
- ☐ MILKY/LACTIC
- ☐ LEMON
- ☐ BUTTERY/CREAMY
- ☐ GRASSY
- ☐ ROBUST
- ☐ HERBAL
- ☐ SKINKY
- ☐ CARAMEL
- ☐ MOLDY/BLUE
- ☐ NUTTY
- ☐ EARTHY

MILK
- ☐ COW
- ☐ SHEEP
- ☐ GOAT
- ☐ RAW
- ☐ OTHER: _____

TEXTURE METER
- RUNNY
- SOFT
- SEMI-SOFT
- SEMI-FIRM
- FIRM
- HARD

NOTES
_____
_____
_____
_____
_____

RATING
☆☆☆☆☆

NAME OF CHEESE _____

FACTORY _____

RIND
- ☐ BLOOMY ☐ WASHED ☐ NATURAL ☐ DRY
  - ☐ WHITE ☐ SALTY ☐ THICK
  - ☐ SOFT   ☐ HARD
  - ☐ FUZZY   ☐ GRITTY

ORIGIN _____

DATE _____

PRICE _____

FLAVORS
- ☐ SALTY
- ☐ SWEET
- ☐ CRYSTALLINE
- ☐ CRUMBLY
- ☐ SHARP/TANGY
- ☐ MILKY/LACTIC
- ☐ LEMON
- ☐ BUTTERY/CREAMY
- ☐ GRASSY
- ☐ ROBUST
- ☐ HERBAL
- ☐ SKINKY
- ☐ CARAMEL
- ☐ MOLDY/BLUE
- ☐ NUTTY
- ☐ EARTHY

MILK
- ☐ COW
- ☐ SHEEP
- ☐ GOAT
- ☐ RAW
- ☐ OTHER: _____
  _____
  _____

TEXTURE METER
- RUNNY
- SOFT
- SEMI-SOFT
- SEMI-FIRM
- FIRM
- HARD

NOTES
_____
_____
_____
_____
_____
_____

RATING
☆ ☆ ☆ ☆ ☆

NAME OF CHEESE _____

FACTORY _____

RIND
- [ ] BLOOMY
- [ ] WASHED
- [ ] NATURAL
- [ ] DRY
  - [ ] WHITE
  - [ ] SALTY
  - [ ] THICK
  - [ ] SOFT
  - [ ] HARD
  - [ ] FUZZY
  - [ ] GRITTY

ORIGIN _____

DATE _____

PRICE _____

FLAVORS
- [ ] SALTY
- [ ] GRASSY
- [ ] SWEET
- [ ] ROBUST
- [ ] CRYSTALLINE
- [ ] HERBAL
- [ ] CRUMBLY
- [ ] SKINKY
- [ ] SHARP/TANGY
- [ ] CARAMEL
- [ ] MILKY/LACTIC
- [ ] MOLDY/BLUE
- [ ] LEMON
- [ ] NUTTY
- [ ] BUTTERY/CREAMY
- [ ] EARTHY

MILK
- [ ] COW
- [ ] SHEEP
- [ ] GOAT
- [ ] RAW
- [ ] OTHER: _____
  _____
  _____

TEXTURE METER
- RUNNY
- SOFT
- SEMI-SOFT
- SEMI-FIRM
- FIRM
- HARD

NOTES
_____
_____
_____
_____
_____
_____

RATING ☆☆☆☆☆

NAME OF CHEESE _____

FACTORY _____

RIND
- [ ] BLOOMY
- [ ] WASHED
- [ ] NATURAL
- [ ] DRY
- [ ] WHITE
- [ ] SALTY
- [ ] THICK
- [ ] SOFT
- [ ] HARD
- [ ] FUZZY
- [ ] GRITTY

ORIGIN _____

DATE _____

PRICE _____

FLAVORS
- [ ] SALTY
- [ ] GRASSY
- [ ] SWEET
- [ ] ROBUST
- [ ] CRYSTALLINE
- [ ] HERBAL
- [ ] CRUMBLY
- [ ] SKINKY
- [ ] SHARP/TANGY
- [ ] CARAMEL
- [ ] MILKY/LACTIC
- [ ] MOLDY/BLUE
- [ ] LEMON
- [ ] NUTTY
- [ ] BUTTERY/CREAMY
- [ ] EARTHY

MILK
- [ ] COW
- [ ] SHEEP
- [ ] GOAT
- [ ] RAW
- [ ] OTHER: _____
  _____
  _____

TEXTURE METER
- RUNNY
- SOFT
- SEMI-SOFT
- SEMI-FIRM
- FIRM
- HARD

NOTES
_____
_____
_____
_____
_____
_____

RATING ☆ ☆ ☆ ☆ ☆

NAME OF CHEESE _____

FACTORY _____

RIND
- [ ] BLOOMY
- [ ] WASHED
- [ ] NATURAL
- [ ] DRY
  - [ ] WHITE
  - [ ] SALTY
  - [ ] THICK
  - [ ] SOFT
  - [ ] HARD
  - [ ] FUZZY
  - [ ] GRITTY

ORIGIN _____

DATE _____

PRICE _____

FLAVORS
- [ ] SALTY
- [ ] SWEET
- [ ] CRYSTALLINE
- [ ] CRUMBLY
- [ ] SHARP/TANGY
- [ ] MILKY/LACTIC
- [ ] LEMON
- [ ] BUTTERY/CREAMY
- [ ] GRASSY
- [ ] ROBUST
- [ ] HERBAL
- [ ] SKINKY
- [ ] CARAMEL
- [ ] MOLDY/BLUE
- [ ] NUTTY
- [ ] EARTHY

MILK
- [ ] COW
- [ ] SHEEP
- [ ] GOAT
- [ ] RAW
- [ ] OTHER: _____
  _____
  _____

TEXTURE METER
- RUNNY
- SOFT
- SEMI-SOFT
- SEMI-FIRM
- FIRM
- HARD

NOTES
_____
_____
_____
_____
_____
_____

RATING
☆ ☆ ☆ ☆ ☆

NAME OF CHEESE _____

FACTORY _____

RIND
- ☐ BLOOMY ☐ WASHED ☐ NATURAL ☐ DRY
  - ☐ WHITE ☐ SALTY ☐ THICK
  - ☐ SOFT ☐ HARD
  - ☐ FUZZY ☐ GRITTY

ORIGIN _____

DATE _____

PRICE _____

FLAVORS
- ☐ SALTY
- ☐ SWEET
- ☐ CRYSTALLINE
- ☐ CRUMBLY
- ☐ SHARP/TANGY
- ☐ MILKY/LACTIC
- ☐ LEMON
- ☐ BUTTERY/CREAMY
- ☐ GRASSY
- ☐ ROBUST
- ☐ HERBAL
- ☐ SKINKY
- ☐ CARAMEL
- ☐ MOLDY/BLUE
- ☐ NUTTY
- ☐ EARTHY

MILK
- ☐ COW
- ☐ SHEEP
- ☐ GOAT
- ☐ RAW
- ☐ OTHER: _____
  - _____
  - _____

TEXTURE METER
- RUNNY
- SOFT
- SEMI-SOFT
- SEMI-FIRM
- FIRM
- HARD

NOTES
_____
_____
_____
_____
_____

RATING
☆ ☆ ☆ ☆ ☆

NAME OF CHEESE _____

FACTORY _____

RIND
- ☐ BLOOMY ☐ WASHED ☐ NATURAL ☐ DRY
  - ☐ WHITE   ☐ SALTY   ☐ THICK
  - ☐ SOFT   ☐ HARD
  - ☐ FUZZY   ☐ GRITTY

ORIGIN _____

DATE _____

PRICE _____

FLAVORS
- ☐ SALTY
- ☐ SWEET
- ☐ CRYSTALLINE
- ☐ CRUMBLY
- ☐ SHARP/TANGY
- ☐ MILKY/LACTIC
- ☐ LEMON
- ☐ BUTTERY/CREAMY
- ☐ GRASSY
- ☐ ROBUST
- ☐ HERBAL
- ☐ SKINKY
- ☐ CARAMEL
- ☐ MOLDY/BLUE
- ☐ NUTTY
- ☐ EARTHY

MILK
- ☐ COW
- ☐ SHEEP
- ☐ GOAT
- ☐ RAW
- ☐ OTHER: _____

TEXTURE METER
- RUNNY
- SOFT
- SEMI-SOFT
- SEMI-FIRM
- FIRM
- HARD

NOTES
_____
_____
_____
_____
_____

RATING ☆ ☆ ☆ ☆ ☆

NAME OF CHEESE _____

FACTORY _____

RIND

- [ ] BLOOMY
- [ ] WASHED
- [ ] NATURAL
- [ ] DRY
  - [ ] WHITE
  - [ ] SALTY
  - [ ] THICK
  - [ ] SOFT
  - [ ] HARD
  - [ ] FUZZY
  - [ ] GRITTY

ORIGIN _____

DATE _____

PRICE _____

FLAVORS

- [ ] SALTY
- [ ] GRASSY
- [ ] SWEET
- [ ] ROBUST
- [ ] CRYSTALLINE
- [ ] HERBAL
- [ ] CRUMBLY
- [ ] SKINKY
- [ ] SHARP/TANGY
- [ ] CARAMEL
- [ ] MILKY/LACTIC
- [ ] MOLDY/BLUE
- [ ] LEMON
- [ ] NUTTY
- [ ] BUTTERY/CREAMY
- [ ] EARTHY

MILK

- [ ] COW
- [ ] SHEEP
- [ ] GOAT
- [ ] RAW
- [ ] OTHER: _____
  _____
  _____

TEXTURE METER

- RUNNY
- SOFT
- SEMI-SOFT
- SEMI-FIRM
- FIRM
- HARD

NOTES

_____
_____
_____
_____
_____
_____

RATING

☆ ☆ ☆ ☆ ☆

NAME OF CHEESE _____

FACTORY _____

RIND
- ☐ BLOOMY ☐ WASHED ☐ NATURAL ☐ DRY
  - ☐ WHITE ☐ SALTY ☐ THICK
  - ☐ SOFT ☐ HARD
  - ☐ FUZZY ☐ GRITTY

ORIGIN _____

DATE _____

PRICE _____

FLAVORS
- ☐ SALTY
- ☐ SWEET
- ☐ CRYSTALLINE
- ☐ CRUMBLY
- ☐ SHARP/TANGY
- ☐ MILKY/LACTIC
- ☐ LEMON
- ☐ BUTTERY/CREAMY
- ☐ GRASSY
- ☐ ROBUST
- ☐ HERBAL
- ☐ SKINKY
- ☐ CARAMEL
- ☐ MOLDY/BLUE
- ☐ NUTTY
- ☐ EARTHY

MILK
- ☐ COW
- ☐ SHEEP
- ☐ GOAT
- ☐ RAW
- ☐ OTHER: _____
  _____
  _____

TEXTURE METER
- RUNNY
- SOFT
- SEMI-SOFT
- SEMI-FIRM
- FIRM
- HARD

NOTES
_____
_____
_____
_____
_____
_____

RATING
☆ ☆ ☆ ☆ ☆

NAME OF CHEESE _____

FACTORY _____

RIND

- ☐ BLOOMY ☐ WASHED ☐ NATURAL ☐ DRY
  - ☐ WHITE   ☐ SALTY   ☐ THICK
  - ☐ SOFT   ☐ HARD
  - ☐ FUZZY   ☐ GRITTY

ORIGIN _____

DATE _____

PRICE _____

FLAVORS

- ☐ SALTY
- ☐ SWEET
- ☐ CRYSTALLINE
- ☐ CRUMBLY
- ☐ SHARP/TANGY
- ☐ MILKY/LACTIC
- ☐ LEMON
- ☐ BUTTERY/CREAMY
- ☐ GRASSY
- ☐ ROBUST
- ☐ HERBAL
- ☐ SKINKY
- ☐ CARAMEL
- ☐ MOLDY/BLUE
- ☐ NUTTY
- ☐ EARTHY

MILK

- ☐ COW
- ☐ SHEEP
- ☐ GOAT
- ☐ RAW
- ☐ OTHER: _____
  _____
  _____

TEXTURE METER

- RUNNY
- SOFT
- SEMI-SOFT
- SEMI-FIRM
- FIRM
- HARD

NOTES

_____
_____
_____
_____
_____
_____

RATING

☆ ☆ ☆ ☆ ☆

NAME OF CHEESE _____

FACTORY _____

RIND
- ☐ BLOOMY   ☐ WASHED   ☐ NATURAL   ☐ DRY
  - ☐ WHITE   ☐ SALTY   ☐ THICK
  - ☐ SOFT   ☐ HARD
  - ☐ FUZZY   ☐ GRITTY

ORIGIN _____

DATE _____

PRICE _____

FLAVORS
- ☐ SALTY   ☐ GRASSY
- ☐ SWEET   ☐ ROBUST
- ☐ CRYSTALLINE   ☐ HERBAL
- ☐ CRUMBLY   ☐ SKINKY
- ☐ SHARP/TANGY   ☐ CARAMEL
- ☐ MILKY/LACTIC   ☐ MOLDY/BLUE
- ☐ LEMON   ☐ NUTTY
- ☐ BUTTERY/CREAMY   ☐ EARTHY

MILK
- ☐ COW
- ☐ SHEEP
- ☐ GOAT
- ☐ RAW
- ☐ OTHER: _____
  _____
  _____

TEXTURE METER
- RUNNY
- SOFT
- SEMI-SOFT
- SEMI-FIRM
- FIRM
- HARD

NOTES
_____
_____
_____
_____
_____

RATING
☆ ☆ ☆ ☆ ☆

NAME OF CHEESE _____

FACTORY _____

RIND
- ☐ BLOOMY ☐ WASHED ☐ NATURAL ☐ DRY
  - ☐ WHITE ☐ SALTY ☐ THICK
  - ☐ SOFT ☐ HARD
  - ☐ FUZZY ☐ GRITTY

ORIGIN _____

DATE _____

PRICE _____

FLAVORS
- ☐ SALTY ☐ GRASSY
- ☐ SWEET ☐ ROBUST
- ☐ CRYSTALLINE ☐ HERBAL
- ☐ CRUMBLY ☐ SKINKY
- ☐ SHARP/TANGY ☐ CARAMEL
- ☐ MILKY/LACTIC ☐ MOLDY/BLUE
- ☐ LEMON ☐ NUTTY
- ☐ BUTTERY/CREAMY ☐ EARTHY

MILK
- ☐ COW
- ☐ SHEEP
- ☐ GOAT
- ☐ RAW
- ☐ OTHER: _____

TEXTURE METER
- RUNNY
- SOFT
- SEMI-SOFT
- SEMI-FIRM
- FIRM
- HARD

NOTES
_____
_____
_____
_____
_____
_____

RATING ☆☆☆☆☆

NAME OF CHEESE _____

FACTORY _____

RIND
- [ ] BLOOMY
  - [ ] WHITE
  - [ ] SOFT
  - [ ] FUZZY
- [ ] WASHED
  - [ ] SALTY
- [ ] NATURAL
  - [ ] THICK
  - [ ] HARD
  - [ ] GRITTY
- [ ] DRY

ORIGIN _____

DATE _____

PRICE _____

FLAVORS
- [ ] SALTY
- [ ] SWEET
- [ ] CRYSTALLINE
- [ ] CRUMBLY
- [ ] SHARP/TANGY
- [ ] MILKY/LACTIC
- [ ] LEMON
- [ ] BUTTERY/CREAMY
- [ ] GRASSY
- [ ] ROBUST
- [ ] HERBAL
- [ ] SKINKY
- [ ] CARAMEL
- [ ] MOLDY/BLUE
- [ ] NUTTY
- [ ] EARTHY

MILK
- [ ] COW
- [ ] SHEEP
- [ ] GOAT
- [ ] RAW
- [ ] OTHER: _____
  _____
  _____

TEXTURE METER
- RUNNY
- SOFT
- SEMI-SOFT
- SEMI-FIRM
- FIRM
- HARD

NOTES
_____
_____
_____
_____
_____
_____

RATING
☆☆☆☆☆

NAME OF CHEESE _____

FACTORY _____

RIND
- ☐ BLOOMY ☐ WASHED ☐ NATURAL ☐ DRY
  - ☐ WHITE   ☐ SALTY   ☐ THICK
  - ☐ SOFT   ☐ HARD
  - ☐ FUZZY   ☐ GRITTY

ORIGIN _____

DATE _____

PRICE _____

FLAVORS
- ☐ SALTY   ☐ GRASSY
- ☐ SWEET   ☐ ROBUST
- ☐ CRYSTALLINE   ☐ HERBAL
- ☐ CRUMBLY   ☐ SKINKY
- ☐ SHARP/TANGY   ☐ CARAMEL
- ☐ MILKY/LACTIC   ☐ MOLDY/BLUE
- ☐ LEMON   ☐ NUTTY
- ☐ BUTTERY/CREAMY ☐ EARTHY

MILK
- ☐ COW
- ☐ SHEEP
- ☐ GOAT
- ☐ RAW
- ☐ OTHER: _____
  _____
  _____

TEXTURE METER
- RUNNY
- SOFT
- SEMI-SOFT
- SEMI-FIRM
- FIRM
- HARD

NOTES
_____
_____
_____
_____
_____
_____

RATING
☆ ☆ ☆ ☆ ☆

NAME OF CHEESE _____

FACTORY _____

RIND
- [ ] BLOOMY
- [ ] WASHED
- [ ] NATURAL
- [ ] DRY
  - [ ] WHITE
  - [ ] SALTY
  - [ ] THICK
  - [ ] SOFT
  - [ ] HARD
  - [ ] FUZZY
  - [ ] GRITTY

ORIGIN _____

DATE _____

PRICE _____

FLAVORS
- [ ] SALTY
- [ ] GRASSY
- [ ] SWEET
- [ ] ROBUST
- [ ] CRYSTALLINE
- [ ] HERBAL
- [ ] CRUMBLY
- [ ] SKINKY
- [ ] SHARP/TANGY
- [ ] CARAMEL
- [ ] MILKY/LACTIC
- [ ] MOLDY/BLUE
- [ ] LEMON
- [ ] NUTTY
- [ ] BUTTERY/CREAMY
- [ ] EARTHY

MILK
- [ ] COW
- [ ] SHEEP
- [ ] GOAT
- [ ] RAW
- [ ] OTHER: _____
  _____
  _____

TEXTURE METER
- RUNNY
- SOFT
- SEMI-SOFT
- SEMI-FIRM
- FIRM
- HARD

NOTES
_____
_____
_____
_____
_____

RATING
☆ ☆ ☆ ☆ ☆

NAME OF CHEESE _____

FACTORY _____

RIND
- [ ] BLOOMY
- [ ] WASHED
- [ ] NATURAL
- [ ] DRY
  - [ ] WHITE
  - [ ] SALTY
  - [ ] THICK
  - [ ] SOFT
  - [ ] HARD
  - [ ] FUZZY
  - [ ] GRITTY

ORIGIN _____

DATE _____

PRICE _____

FLAVORS
- [ ] SALTY
- [ ] GRASSY
- [ ] SWEET
- [ ] ROBUST
- [ ] CRYSTALLINE
- [ ] HERBAL
- [ ] CRUMBLY
- [ ] SKINKY
- [ ] SHARP/TANGY
- [ ] CARAMEL
- [ ] MILKY/LACTIC
- [ ] MOLDY/BLUE
- [ ] LEMON
- [ ] NUTTY
- [ ] BUTTERY/CREAMY
- [ ] EARTHY

MILK
- [ ] COW
- [ ] SHEEP
- [ ] GOAT
- [ ] RAW
- [ ] OTHER: _____
  _____
  _____

TEXTURE METER
- RUNNY
- SOFT
- SEMI-SOFT
- SEMI-FIRM
- FIRM
- HARD

NOTES
_____
_____
_____
_____
_____

RATING
☆ ☆ ☆ ☆ ☆

NAME OF CHEESE _____

FACTORY _____

RIND
- [ ] BLOOMY
- [ ] WASHED
- [ ] NATURAL
- [ ] DRY
  - [ ] WHITE
  - [ ] SALTY
  - [ ] THICK
  - [ ] SOFT
  - [ ] HARD
  - [ ] FUZZY
  - [ ] GRITTY

ORIGIN _____

DATE _____

PRICE _____

FLAVORS
- [ ] SALTY
- [ ] GRASSY
- [ ] SWEET
- [ ] ROBUST
- [ ] CRYSTALLINE
- [ ] HERBAL
- [ ] CRUMBLY
- [ ] SKINKY
- [ ] SHARP/TANGY
- [ ] CARAMEL
- [ ] MILKY/LACTIC
- [ ] MOLDY/BLUE
- [ ] LEMON
- [ ] NUTTY
- [ ] BUTTERY/CREAMY
- [ ] EARTHY

MILK
- [ ] COW
- [ ] SHEEP
- [ ] GOAT
- [ ] RAW
- [ ] OTHER: _____
  _____
  _____

TEXTURE METER
- RUNNY
- SOFT
- SEMI-SOFT
- SEMI-FIRM
- FIRM
- HARD

NOTES
_____
_____
_____
_____
_____

RATING
☆ ☆ ☆ ☆ ☆

NAME OF CHEESE _____

FACTORY _____

RIND
- ☐ BLOOMY ☐ WASHED ☐ NATURAL ☐ DRY
  - ☐ WHITE   ☐ SALTY   ☐ THICK
  - ☐ SOFT   ☐ HARD
  - ☐ FUZZY   ☐ GRITTY

ORIGIN _____

DATE _____

PRICE _____

FLAVORS
- ☐ SALTY
- ☐ SWEET
- ☐ CRYSTALLINE
- ☐ CRUMBLY
- ☐ SHARP/TANGY
- ☐ MILKY/LACTIC
- ☐ LEMON
- ☐ BUTTERY/CREAMY
- ☐ GRASSY
- ☐ ROBUST
- ☐ HERBAL
- ☐ SKINKY
- ☐ CARAMEL
- ☐ MOLDY/BLUE
- ☐ NUTTY
- ☐ EARTHY

MILK
- ☐ COW
- ☐ SHEEP
- ☐ GOAT
- ☐ RAW
- ☐ OTHER: _____
  _____
  _____

TEXTURE METER
- RUNNY
- SOFT
- SEMI-SOFT
- SEMI-FIRM
- FIRM
- HARD

NOTES
_____
_____
_____
_____
_____
_____

RATING ☆☆☆☆☆

NAME OF CHEESE _____

FACTORY _____

RIND

- [ ] BLOOMY
- [ ] WASHED
- [ ] NATURAL
- [ ] DRY
- [ ] WHITE
- [ ] SALTY
- [ ] THICK
- [ ] SOFT
- [ ] HARD
- [ ] FUZZY
- [ ] GRITTY

ORIGIN _____

DATE _____

PRICE _____

FLAVORS

- [ ] SALTY
- [ ] GRASSY
- [ ] SWEET
- [ ] ROBUST
- [ ] CRYSTALLINE
- [ ] HERBAL
- [ ] CRUMBLY
- [ ] SKINKY
- [ ] SHARP/TANGY
- [ ] CARAMEL
- [ ] MILKY/LACTIC
- [ ] MOLDY/BLUE
- [ ] LEMON
- [ ] NUTTY
- [ ] BUTTERY/CREAMY
- [ ] EARTHY

MILK

- [ ] COW
- [ ] SHEEP
- [ ] GOAT
- [ ] RAW
- [ ] OTHER: _____

TEXTURE METER

- RUNNY
- SOFT
- SEMI-SOFT
- SEMI-FIRM
- FIRM
- HARD

NOTES

_____
_____
_____
_____
_____
_____

RATING
☆☆☆☆☆

NAME OF CHEESE _____

FACTORY _____

RIND
- ☐ BLOOMY ☐ WASHED ☐ NATURAL ☐ DRY
  - ☐ WHITE ☐ SALTY ☐ THICK
  - ☐ SOFT ☐ HARD
  - ☐ FUZZY ☐ GRITTY

ORIGIN _____

DATE _____

PRICE _____

FLAVORS
- ☐ SALTY ☐ GRASSY
- ☐ SWEET ☐ ROBUST
- ☐ CRYSTALLINE ☐ HERBAL
- ☐ CRUMBLY ☐ SKINKY
- ☐ SHARP/TANGY ☐ CARAMEL
- ☐ MILKY/LACTIC ☐ MOLDY/BLUE
- ☐ LEMON ☐ NUTTY
- ☐ BUTTERY/CREAMY ☐ EARTHY

MILK
- ☐ COW
- ☐ SHEEP
- ☐ GOAT
- ☐ RAW
- ☐ OTHER: _____
  _____
  _____

TEXTURE METER
- RUNNY
- SOFT
- SEMI-SOFT
- SEMI-FIRM
- FIRM
- HARD

NOTES
_____
_____
_____
_____
_____

RATING ☆☆☆☆☆

NAME OF CHEESE _____

FACTORY _____

RIND
- [ ] BLOOMY
- [ ] WASHED
- [ ] NATURAL
- [ ] DRY
  - [ ] WHITE
  - [ ] SALTY
  - [ ] THICK
  - [ ] SOFT
  - [ ] HARD
  - [ ] FUZZY
  - [ ] GRITTY

ORIGIN _____

DATE _____

PRICE _____

FLAVORS
- [ ] SALTY
- [ ] GRASSY
- [ ] SWEET
- [ ] ROBUST
- [ ] CRYSTALLINE
- [ ] HERBAL
- [ ] CRUMBLY
- [ ] SKINKY
- [ ] SHARP/TANGY
- [ ] CARAMEL
- [ ] MILKY/LACTIC
- [ ] MOLDY/BLUE
- [ ] LEMON
- [ ] NUTTY
- [ ] BUTTERY/CREAMY
- [ ] EARTHY

MILK
- [ ] COW
- [ ] SHEEP
- [ ] GOAT
- [ ] RAW
- [ ] OTHER: _____
_____
_____

TEXTURE METER
- RUNNY
- SOFT
- SEMI-SOFT
- SEMI-FIRM
- FIRM
- HARD

NOTES
_____
_____
_____
_____
_____
_____

RATING
☆ ☆ ☆ ☆ ☆

NAME OF CHEESE _____

FACTORY _____

RIND
- ☐ BLOOMY ☐ WASHED ☐ NATURAL ☐ DRY
  - ☐ WHITE   ☐ SALTY   ☐ THICK
  - ☐ SOFT   ☐ HARD
  - ☐ FUZZY   ☐ GRITTY

ORIGIN _____

DATE _____

PRICE _____

FLAVORS
- ☐ SALTY   ☐ GRASSY
- ☐ SWEET   ☐ ROBUST
- ☐ CRYSTALLINE   ☐ HERBAL
- ☐ CRUMBLY   ☐ SKINKY
- ☐ SHARP/TANGY   ☐ CARAMEL
- ☐ MILKY/LACTIC   ☐ MOLDY/BLUE
- ☐ LEMON   ☐ NUTTY
- ☐ BUTTERY/CREAMY   ☐ EARTHY

MILK
- ☐ COW
- ☐ SHEEP
- ☐ GOAT
- ☐ RAW
- ☐ OTHER: _____
  _____
  _____

TEXTURE METER
- RUNNY
- SOFT
- SEMI-SOFT
- SEMI-FIRM
- FIRM
- HARD

NOTES
_____
_____
_____
_____
_____

RATING
☆ ☆ ☆ ☆ ☆

NAME OF CHEESE _____

FACTORY _____

RIND
- ☐ BLOOMY   ☐ WASHED   ☐ NATURAL   ☐ DRY
  - ☐ WHITE   ☐ SALTY   ☐ THICK
  - ☐ SOFT   ☐ HARD
  - ☐ FUZZY   ☐ GRITTY

ORIGIN _____

DATE _____

PRICE _____

FLAVORS
- ☐ SALTY   ☐ GRASSY
- ☐ SWEET   ☐ ROBUST
- ☐ CRYSTALLINE   ☐ HERBAL
- ☐ CRUMBLY   ☐ SKINKY
- ☐ SHARP/TANGY   ☐ CARAMEL
- ☐ MILKY/LACTIC   ☐ MOLDY/BLUE
- ☐ LEMON   ☐ NUTTY
- ☐ BUTTERY/CREAMY   ☐ EARTHY

MILK
- ☐ COW
- ☐ SHEEP
- ☐ GOAT
- ☐ RAW
- ☐ OTHER: _____
  _____
  _____

TEXTURE METER
- RUNNY
- SOFT
- SEMI-SOFT
- SEMI-FIRM
- FIRM
- HARD

NOTES
_____
_____
_____
_____
_____

RATING ☆☆☆☆☆

NAME OF CHEESE _____

FACTORY _____

RIND
- [ ] BLOOMY   [ ] WASHED   [ ] NATURAL   [ ] DRY
  - [ ] WHITE   [ ] SALTY   [ ] THICK
  - [ ] SOFT   [ ] HARD
  - [ ] FUZZY   [ ] GRITTY

ORIGIN _____

DATE _____

PRICE _____

FLAVORS
- [ ] SALTY
- [ ] SWEET
- [ ] CRYSTALLINE
- [ ] CRUMBLY
- [ ] SHARP/TANGY
- [ ] MILKY/LACTIC
- [ ] LEMON
- [ ] BUTTERY/CREAMY
- [ ] GRASSY
- [ ] ROBUST
- [ ] HERBAL
- [ ] SKINKY
- [ ] CARAMEL
- [ ] MOLDY/BLUE
- [ ] NUTTY
- [ ] EARTHY

MILK
- [ ] COW
- [ ] SHEEP
- [ ] GOAT
- [ ] RAW
- [ ] OTHER: _____
  _____
  _____

TEXTURE METER
- RUNNY
- SOFT
- SEMI-SOFT
- SEMI-FIRM
- FIRM
- HARD

NOTES
_____
_____
_____
_____
_____
_____

RATING
☆ ☆ ☆ ☆ ☆

NAME OF CHEESE _____

FACTORY _____

RIND
- ☐ BLOOMY ☐ WASHED ☐ NATURAL ☐ DRY
  - ☐ WHITE ☐ SALTY ☐ THICK
  - ☐ SOFT   ☐ HARD
  - ☐ FUZZY   ☐ GRITTY

ORIGIN _____

DATE _____

PRICE _____

FLAVORS
- ☐ SALTY   ☐ GRASSY
- ☐ SWEET   ☐ ROBUST
- ☐ CRYSTALLINE   ☐ HERBAL
- ☐ CRUMBLY   ☐ SKINKY
- ☐ SHARP/TANGY   ☐ CARAMEL
- ☐ MILKY/LACTIC   ☐ MOLDY/BLUE
- ☐ LEMON   ☐ NUTTY
- ☐ BUTTERY/CREAMY ☐ EARTHY

MILK
- ☐ COW
- ☐ SHEEP
- ☐ GOAT
- ☐ RAW
- ☐ OTHER: _____

TEXTURE METER
- RUNNY
- SOFT
- SEMI-SOFT
- SEMI-FIRM
- FIRM
- HARD

NOTES
_____
_____
_____
_____
_____

RATING
☆ ☆ ☆ ☆ ☆

NAME OF CHEESE _____

FACTORY _____

RIND
- ☐ BLOOMY ☐ WASHED ☐ NATURAL ☐ DRY
  - ☐ WHITE ☐ SALTY ☐ THICK
  - ☐ SOFT ☐ HARD
  - ☐ FUZZY ☐ GRITTY

ORIGIN _____

DATE _____

PRICE _____

FLAVORS
- ☐ SALTY
- ☐ SWEET
- ☐ CRYSTALLINE
- ☐ CRUMBLY
- ☐ SHARP/TANGY
- ☐ MILKY/LACTIC
- ☐ LEMON
- ☐ BUTTERY/CREAMY
- ☐ GRASSY
- ☐ ROBUST
- ☐ HERBAL
- ☐ SKINKY
- ☐ CARAMEL
- ☐ MOLDY/BLUE
- ☐ NUTTY
- ☐ EARTHY

MILK
- ☐ COW
- ☐ SHEEP
- ☐ GOAT
- ☐ RAW
- ☐ OTHER: _____
  _____
  _____

TEXTURE METER
- RUNNY
- SOFT
- SEMI-SOFT
- SEMI-FIRM
- FIRM
- HARD

NOTES
_____
_____
_____
_____
_____
_____

RATING
☆ ☆ ☆ ☆ ☆

NAME OF CHEESE _____

FACTORY _____

RIND
- [ ] BLOOMY
- [ ] WASHED
- [ ] NATURAL
- [ ] DRY
  - [ ] WHITE
  - [ ] SALTY
  - [ ] THICK
  - [ ] SOFT
  - [ ] HARD
  - [ ] FUZZY
  - [ ] GRITTY

ORIGIN _____

DATE _____

PRICE _____

FLAVORS
- [ ] SALTY
- [ ] GRASSY
- [ ] SWEET
- [ ] ROBUST
- [ ] CRYSTALLINE
- [ ] HERBAL
- [ ] CRUMBLY
- [ ] SKINKY
- [ ] SHARP/TANGY
- [ ] CARAMEL
- [ ] MILKY/LACTIC
- [ ] MOLDY/BLUE
- [ ] LEMON
- [ ] NUTTY
- [ ] BUTTERY/CREAMY
- [ ] EARTHY

MILK
- [ ] COW
- [ ] SHEEP
- [ ] GOAT
- [ ] RAW
- [ ] OTHER: _____

TEXTURE METER
- RUNNY
- SOFT
- SEMI-SOFT
- SEMI-FIRM
- FIRM
- HARD

NOTES
_____
_____
_____
_____
_____

RATING
☆ ☆ ☆ ☆ ☆

NAME OF CHEESE _____

FACTORY _____

RIND
- [ ] BLOOMY
- [ ] WASHED
- [ ] NATURAL
- [ ] DRY
  - [ ] WHITE
  - [ ] SALTY
  - [ ] THICK
  - [ ] SOFT
  - [ ] HARD
  - [ ] FUZZY
  - [ ] GRITTY

ORIGIN _____

DATE _____

PRICE _____

FLAVORS
- [ ] SALTY
- [ ] GRASSY
- [ ] SWEET
- [ ] ROBUST
- [ ] CRYSTALLINE
- [ ] HERBAL
- [ ] CRUMBLY
- [ ] SKINKY
- [ ] SHARP/TANGY
- [ ] CARAMEL
- [ ] MILKY/LACTIC
- [ ] MOLDY/BLUE
- [ ] LEMON
- [ ] NUTTY
- [ ] BUTTERY/CREAMY
- [ ] EARTHY

MILK
- [ ] COW
- [ ] SHEEP
- [ ] GOAT
- [ ] RAW
- [ ] OTHER: _____
  _____
  _____

TEXTURE METER
- RUNNY
- SOFT
- SEMI-SOFT
- SEMI-FIRM
- FIRM
- HARD

NOTES
_____
_____
_____
_____
_____

RATING
☆ ☆ ☆ ☆ ☆

NAME OF CHEESE _____

FACTORY _____

RIND
- [ ] BLOOMY
- [ ] WASHED
- [ ] NATURAL
- [ ] DRY
- [ ] WHITE
- [ ] SALTY
- [ ] THICK
- [ ] SOFT
- [ ] HARD
- [ ] FUZZY
- [ ] GRITTY

ORIGIN _____

DATE _____

PRICE _____

FLAVORS
- [ ] SALTY
- [ ] SWEET
- [ ] CRYSTALLINE
- [ ] CRUMBLY
- [ ] SHARP/TANGY
- [ ] MILKY/LACTIC
- [ ] LEMON
- [ ] BUTTERY/CREAMY
- [ ] GRASSY
- [ ] ROBUST
- [ ] HERBAL
- [ ] SKINKY
- [ ] CARAMEL
- [ ] MOLDY/BLUE
- [ ] NUTTY
- [ ] EARTHY

MILK
- [ ] COW
- [ ] SHEEP
- [ ] GOAT
- [ ] RAW
- [ ] OTHER: _____

TEXTURE METER
- RUNNY
- SOFT
- SEMI-SOFT
- SEMI-FIRM
- FIRM
- HARD

NOTES
_____
_____
_____
_____
_____

RATING
☆ ☆ ☆ ☆ ☆

NAME OF CHEESE _____

FACTORY _____

RIND
- ☐ BLOOMY ☐ WASHED ☐ NATURAL ☐ DRY
  - ☐ WHITE ☐ SALTY ☐ THICK
  - ☐ SOFT   ☐ HARD
  - ☐ FUZZY   ☐ GRITTY

ORIGIN _____

DATE _____

PRICE _____

FLAVORS
- ☐ SALTY
- ☐ SWEET
- ☐ CRYSTALLINE
- ☐ CRUMBLY
- ☐ SHARP/TANGY
- ☐ MILKY/LACTIC
- ☐ LEMON
- ☐ BUTTERY/CREAMY
- ☐ GRASSY
- ☐ ROBUST
- ☐ HERBAL
- ☐ SKINKY
- ☐ CARAMEL
- ☐ MOLDY/BLUE
- ☐ NUTTY
- ☐ EARTHY

MILK
- ☐ COW
- ☐ SHEEP
- ☐ GOAT
- ☐ RAW
- ☐ OTHER: _____
  _____
  _____

TEXTURE METER
- RUNNY
- SOFT
- SEMI-SOFT
- SEMI-FIRM
- FIRM
- HARD

NOTES
_____
_____
_____
_____
_____

RATING
☆ ☆ ☆ ☆ ☆

NAME OF CHEESE _____

FACTORY _____

RIND

- ☐ BLOOMY ☐ WASHED ☐ NATURAL ☐ DRY
  - ☐ WHITE ☐ SALTY ☐ THICK
  - ☐ SOFT   ☐ HARD
  - ☐ FUZZY   ☐ GRITTY

ORIGIN _____

DATE _____

PRICE _____

FLAVORS

- ☐ SALTY
- ☐ SWEET
- ☐ CRYSTALLINE
- ☐ CRUMBLY
- ☐ SHARP/TANGY
- ☐ MILKY/LACTIC
- ☐ LEMON
- ☐ BUTTERY/CREAMY
- ☐ GRASSY
- ☐ ROBUST
- ☐ HERBAL
- ☐ SKINKY
- ☐ CARAMEL
- ☐ MOLDY/BLUE
- ☐ NUTTY
- ☐ EARTHY

MILK

- ☐ COW
- ☐ SHEEP
- ☐ GOAT
- ☐ RAW
- ☐ OTHER: _____
  _____
  _____

TEXTURE METER

- RUNNY
- SOFT
- SEMI-SOFT
- SEMI-FIRM
- FIRM
- HARD

NOTES

_____
_____
_____
_____
_____

RATING

☆ ☆ ☆ ☆ ☆

NAME OF CHEESE _____

FACTORY _____

RIND

- [ ] BLOOMY ☐ WASHED ☐ NATURAL ☐ DRY
  - [ ] WHITE ☐ SALTY ☐ THICK
  - [ ] SOFT ☐ HARD
  - [ ] FUZZY ☐ GRITTY

ORIGIN _____

DATE _____

PRICE _____

FLAVORS

- [ ] SALTY
- [ ] SWEET
- [ ] CRYSTALLINE
- [ ] CRUMBLY
- [ ] SHARP/TANGY
- [ ] MILKY/LACTIC
- [ ] LEMON
- [ ] BUTTERY/CREAMY
- [ ] GRASSY
- [ ] ROBUST
- [ ] HERBAL
- [ ] SKINKY
- [ ] CARAMEL
- [ ] MOLDY/BLUE
- [ ] NUTTY
- [ ] EARTHY

MILK

- [ ] COW
- [ ] SHEEP
- [ ] GOAT
- [ ] RAW
- [ ] OTHER: _____
  _____
  _____

TEXTURE METER

- RUNNY
- SOFT
- SEMI-SOFT
- SEMI-FIRM
- FIRM
- HARD

NOTES

_____
_____
_____
_____
_____
_____

RATING

☆ ☆ ☆ ☆ ☆

NAME OF CHEESE _____

FACTORY _____

RIND

- [ ] BLOOMY
- [ ] WASHED
- [ ] NATURAL
- [ ] DRY
- [ ] WHITE
- [ ] SALTY
- [ ] THICK
- [ ] SOFT
- [ ] HARD
- [ ] FUZZY
- [ ] GRITTY

ORIGIN _____

DATE _____

PRICE _____

FLAVORS

- [ ] SALTY
- [ ] SWEET
- [ ] CRYSTALLINE
- [ ] CRUMBLY
- [ ] SHARP/TANGY
- [ ] MILKY/LACTIC
- [ ] LEMON
- [ ] BUTTERY/CREAMY
- [ ] GRASSY
- [ ] ROBUST
- [ ] HERBAL
- [ ] SKINKY
- [ ] CARAMEL
- [ ] MOLDY/BLUE
- [ ] NUTTY
- [ ] EARTHY

MILK

- [ ] COW
- [ ] SHEEP
- [ ] GOAT
- [ ] RAW
- [ ] OTHER: _____
  _____
  _____

TEXTURE METER

- RUNNY
- SOFT
- SEMI-SOFT
- SEMI-FIRM
- FIRM
- HARD

NOTES

_____
_____
_____
_____
_____

RATING ☆☆☆☆☆

NAME OF CHEESE _____

FACTORY _____

RIND

- ☐ BLOOMY ☐ WASHED ☐ NATURAL ☐ DRY
  - ☐ WHITE ☐ SALTY ☐ THICK
  - ☐ SOFT   ☐ HARD
  - ☐ FUZZY   ☐ GRITTY

ORIGIN _____

DATE _____

PRICE _____

FLAVORS

- ☐ SALTY   ☐ GRASSY
- ☐ SWEET   ☐ ROBUST
- ☐ CRYSTALLINE   ☐ HERBAL
- ☐ CRUMBLY   ☐ SKINKY
- ☐ SHARP/TANGY   ☐ CARAMEL
- ☐ MILKY/LACTIC   ☐ MOLDY/BLUE
- ☐ LEMON   ☐ NUTTY
- ☐ BUTTERY/CREAMY ☐ EARTHY

MILK

- ☐ COW
- ☐ SHEEP
- ☐ GOAT
- ☐ RAW
- ☐ OTHER:
  _____
  _____
  _____

TEXTURE METER

- RUNNY
- SOFT
- SEMI-SOFT
- SEMI-FIRM
- FIRM
- HARD

NOTES

_____
_____
_____
_____
_____

RATING

☆ ☆ ☆ ☆ ☆

www.ingramcontent.com/pod-product-compliance
Lightning Source LLC
Chambersburg PA
CBHW081155070526
44583CB00021B/2847